BREAK AWAY

BREAK AWAY

DR. FREDERICK ABELES

Published by Cluster One Media
587 Virginia Avenue
Atlanta, Georgia 30306

Break Away: The New Method for Treating Headaches, Migraines and TMJ without Medication / Dr. Frederick Abeles – 1st edition

Printed in the United States of America

Library of Congress Cataloging-in-Publication Data is available

ISBN: 978-0-9864359-0-4

Cover design by Jeff Abeles

To my loving parents, Mort and Jeanne, my amazing wife, Rhona, and my beautiful children, Jennifer and Jeffrey.

CONTENTS

Foreword

Foreword by Dr. William Dickerson – CEO and founder of the Las Vegas Institute for Advanced Dental Studies

Over 9000 dentists from all over the world have attended at least one of the courses at LVI in its 20 years of existence. However, few have taken as many and have kept up with the evolution of this area of dentistry like Dr. Fred Abeles. I was so impressed with his character and passion that I asked him to join our clinical instructor team many years ago and to become a regional director to help spread this important message later.

His passion and enthusiasm has given him the ability to stir the emotions of those he has spoken to about the importance of occlusion (the bite) in dentistry. Dr. Abeles is one of the most prolific lamplighters in this area of our profession that I know and this book exemplifies that as his sincere concern about people and their well-being is dripping from every page.

Some of you may be wondering why your bite matters. What's the big deal? It matters because our physiology dictates it. When our teeth occlude thousands of times a day, the sensory input is sent to our brain from the periodontal ligament that surrounds your teeth through the trigeminal nerve. When you consider that more than half of the total neural input to our brain comes from the trigeminal nerve, clearly nature has placed a great deal of importance on the sensory information coming from this region.

With so much neural input it must go to some very important structures. So what is innervated by the trigeminal nerve?

- The teeth
- The periodontal ligament which connects the teeth to the jaws
- The muscles that move the jaw
- The muscle that tenses the ear drum
- The muscle that opens and closes the Eustachian tubes
- The lining of the sinuses
- Some of the innervation to the tongue
- The jaw joints or TM Joints
- The control of the blood flow to the anterior 2/3 of the brain via the dura mater

When the teeth come together, this sensory feedback, which is called proprioception, is carried back to the brain stem where reflexes are established to either relax the neuromusculature when the occlusion is balanced and in harmony, or to cause an immediate shift to avoid a noxious input, when it is not.

Some of you reading this may have experienced an acute form of this. If the noxious stimulus is temporary, e.g. biting on something unexpectedly hard in your food, the avoidance reflex prevents immediate injury. However when the noxious stimulus is chronic such an occlusal interference from a 'high' filling or crown or a bad bite, the reflexes designed to protect become harmful.

The avoidance affects not only the immediate posture of the jaw but as that shifts, other compensating reflexes affect the head, neck and ultimately total body posture which leads to fatigue and the development of anatomical changes and chronic pain. The trigeminal nerve is also one of the major pain-signaling structures of the brain.

Eliminating interferences in function is a critical part of the understanding and treatment of occlusion. Interferences create noxious stimuli that can result in not just fracture, mobility or sensitive teeth; it can also create an avoidance effect that moves the mandible to a pathologic position to avoid the noxious stimuli. That pathologic position can become a serious pain-causing problem.

The brain spends over 40% of its daily energy deciphering the impulses created by this nerve and the trigeminal and facial nerves account for over 50% of head function. So when your bite is off, your trigeminal complex can easily become overloaded causing symptoms like facial pain, headaches, even migraines.

Occlusion affects so many far-reaching things. Developmental growth conditions during childhood or improper orthodontic and dental treatment can lead to a retruded bite (the jaw too far back). This can cause a postural change to the position of the head - forward head posture - that can affect the muscles of the head, neck and back and lead to chronic pain and TMD (temporal mandibular disorder). It's called the top block effect, where a bite issue can descend down the body creating problems that would otherwise not seem to be associated with the bite, especially the cervical (neck) complex.

In fact, a more appropriate term that TMD is CCDM (Cranio Cervical Mandibular Dysfunction). If we build a bite that is not in physiologic harmony, then it can lead to hypertonic muscles that create chronic pain.

One area that is very much overlooked in our profession is the relationship of the occlusion and muscle disharmony and the effect that has on obstructive sleep apnea in our patients. Not to be an alarmist, but not understanding the relationship of occlusion in this matter can actually have a dentist create OSA and the serious problems associated with it, even death.

Why is there confusion? This is mainly based on a lack of knowledge about the physiological component of the occlusion system. Tradition has created an educational base that ignores this important and critical aspect of occlusion. There is little science to back up the traditional teachings of occlusion but just because something has been taught for a long time does not make it true or accurate. Columbus said, "Even if 1000 people believe something is foolish, it is still foolish".

The medical world uses tools to measure the body's performance for diagnostic purposes, like EEG's, EKG's and EMG's. For some reason, dentistry really never measured the neurological and muscular function of the biting system. Back in the days when the original concepts were developed, the biomedical tools to measure the physiologic response of the body did not exist.

Like medicine, we had to wait until the physiologic measuring tools were developed but that time is now here. Unlike medicine, much of dentistry ignores the measurement of physiology and it is time that dentistry caught up. The dentistry Dr. Abeles talks about in this book has done just that.

The principles discussed in this book can quantify the neutral, balanced and rested position using EMG's and tools to help us reach a physiologic state to determine the best position from which to build the bite, which is in harmony with that patient's physiology. It's really actually quite easy and has been used in many facets of medicine for years.

What we are finding is that everyone who is exposed to this concept completely understands the logic and physiologic science that supports this type of dentistry. Like Dr. Abeles, they are convinced that it's the best path for their patients and themselves. There are many personal stories of dentists who have had their own bites corrected using this approach with life changing results.

What most all dentists agree on is that occlusion is important. However, one school of thought is the 'psychosocial model', which claims occlusion doesn't have anything to do with TMD and that it's all in their head. Basically the patient is crazy. It's just ludicrous to think that TMD is unrelated to the bite.

There is an organized effort, by some insurance consultant dentists, to attempt to make this model the standard of care for obvious reasons. If it's not caused by the bite, they don't have to pay for it. It's this philosophy that has patients using pills to help mask the pain. Dr. Abeles has brilliantly exposed the problems and long term effects of this type of treatment.

Occlusion *always* matters, yet 90% or more of dentists just restore the bite where the patient currently bites. If they are asymptomatic, then that may be fine. But one restoration can change the bite and end up causing problems. Dr. Abeles explains in this book how the loss of the hard tissue vertical posterior stop (the teeth) can cause some serious problems, even though the dentist thinks they are building the bite in the existing position. Even cosmetic restorations done on your front teeth can interfere with your natural chew cycle causing not only breakage of the restorations, but avoidance of the interference and that can lead to TMD symptoms.

That's why it's critical for a dentist to understand the principles of occlusion even though they may not want to treat pain patients, because what they do may actually *create* a pain patient. The biggest problem out there is that dentists can't diagnose what they can't see and they can't see what they don't know. Most dentists are unaware of the obvious signs of occlusion disharmony or the symptoms that indicate a TMD issue.

Wear facets (the edges of the teeth have been worn down), exostosis (excess boney growth around the jaw), abfractions (notches in your tooth at the gum line), loss of vertical (the distance between your nose and chin) and many other common problems that patients exhibit are all indications of occlusal disharmony. If they tell you that the notches and sensitivity at the gum line are due to toothbrush abrasion, they don't understand the importance of occlusion.

Your dentist should also palpate the muscles to determine indications of muscle disharmony. Most dentists don't know the right questions to ask of the patient to determine if they have other symptoms due to a bite issue. They are unaware of the cervical (neck) connection to the bite.

Knowledge is the key to being able to do the best for their patients, and unfortunately, the majority of dentists are lacking in post graduate education. Many stop learning after dental school and yet dental school is really just a license to learn more about dentistry.

Dr. Abeles gives you the tools in this book - what to look for and what questions to ask in order to find the right dentist for your problems.

I want to thank Dr. Abeles for presenting this important subject in a direct, interesting and logical manner that everyone can understand. Please, read this book from cover to cover so you can learn for yourself what might be the problem to your chronic pain or the pain of a loved one.

Let this be the first step to a life-changing journey that will eliminate a lifetime of pain and provide a healthy, longer, happier life. I know that there is a solution to your problem and hope you find the path that can lead you to that resolution and a wonderful life. That is my wish for everyone.

William G. Dickerson, DDS, FAACD, LVIM

Introduction

WAKING UP AT three in the morning, in pain, wondering *why* you're in pain and why no one can figure out how to make the pain stop, is a horrible feeling and unfortunately all too common for many of us.

Chronic, persistent pain wears us down physically and emotionally. Our zest for life diminishes. Our energy is depleted. We can't be at the top of our game when there's pain lurking in the background all the time.

For many of us, after seeing numerous doctors and trying numerous remedies we receive these chilling words that can become a life sentence... "Just learn to live with it."

Or we're told it's, "all in our head" and here's some anti-depressants or anti-anxiety medications to take. Here's a little hint: When your doctor tells you to just live with your pain, they probably have not made a definitive diagnosis and don't know what to do for you, so "Here's some pills to take." Sound familiar?

Many times within three minutes of a new patient sitting down in my private office for a consultation with me, they burst into tears. And I hop up to grab a box of Kleenex for them. Why so? Clearly, their lives are not working for them as they desire or dreamed. They can't be there for their spouse as they want. They can't be there for their kids as they want. They miss days at work.

Pain can take away a lot of the little things in our life we took for granted, like showing up for our loved ones to give them our best. And feeling like ourselves before we were living with chronic pain. You know... the old me that was happy and full of energy.

If you can relate to anything I just wrote, then you know what I mean. There are so many, many people living with chronic pain, headaches, migraines, neck pain, ear pain, jaw joint pain and more.

No one has been able to help them. No one has been able to take their pain away. No one has been able to give them their life back. Instead they wind up with a bag full of pills that "stopped working" or "make me feel drowsy".

If we live with our pain long enough, we *will* need anti-depressants because the pain will wear us down, suck out our life energy and we'll actually become physically depressed. Many of our patients have some form of depression whether it has been diagnosed or not. Chronic pain will wreak havoc with our life in many ways.

So, I would like to abolish your 'life sentence'. I would like to challenge you to find the right knowledge, the right help – to reclaim your life and your happiness. If this sounds good to you, you've come to the right place.

I think it's important at the outset to share with you why I wrote this book. It's certainly not for fame and fortune. Most authors never get wide distribution. Their book never makes it to the masses. I predict the same result here.

But, we are doing some amazing things in our practice for a lot of folks. Not to exaggerate or hype anything and certainly not to try to impress you – we are literally changing people's lives.

Since there's a very good chance I'll never have the opportunity to meet you in person, I felt if I could at least share a glimpse of what we do, some insight into why we do it and how it's helping people recover from so many failed attempts at defeating their pain – it would be of benefit to you.

From my standpoint, if I help just one individual reading this book, to change their life for the better, it will have been worth the time and effort to create it.

So who am I and why should you listen to me?

Well, at the risk of boring you to tears – here's a little of my story. And, I'm going to share some of the important lessons I learned along the way that are relevant to you and your condition. So hang with me.

I was born and raised in Altoona, Pennsylvania. In case you never heard of Altoona, its home to Boyer's Mallo Cups, the Slinky and the Horseshoe Curve. If you haven't heard of those, well, the actor George Burns used to talk about Altoona all the time. In case you haven't heard of George Burns, then you're a youngster. Let's move on.

I had the two best parents in the whole world and an older, wiser sister. I excelled academically in high school with no effort whatsoever. I graduated Altoona High School in 1968.

I went on to Washington and Jefferson College, W&J, the third oldest college in the nation, founded in 1781. It had a superb reputation as a small, private school with a fantastic ratio of professors to students. In those days, if you just graduated from W&J, you were a shoe-in to medical, dental or law school.

My first semester away from home was awesome. I went to classes. I studied the same way I did in high school where I got mostly all 'A's and a few 'B's - which means, I virtually never studied and goofed off a lot. Man, college was fun!

One small problem. At the end of my first semester I wound up with a grade point average of 0.3. You read that correctly... 0.3.

To this day, I hold the record for the *lowest* grade point average ever in the history of W&J for someone who actually graduated. Cool. Let me explain...

When we came back to school after the fall break to register for the second semester, I came back with another buddy of mine from my home town, Gordy C. who was a friend since we were little kids.

Gordy and I both walked up to the registration desk where you signed in and also received slips that showed what courses you were going to take that semester. Gordy was directly in front of me in the line.

He also had a terrible grade point average, but it was over double what mine was. He turned to me and informed me he had flunked out of college and was not being admitted to the winter session. Again, his GPA was twice as high as mine (which still sucked).

I cannot ever share with you the panic and terror I felt at that moment, knowing that my GPA was way less than Gordy's and he was toast. I thought for sure I had already flunked out of college after my first semester.

Well, I walked up to the desk, they handed me my slips and I was registered for all my winter semester courses! Then they gave me a letter. I was to report to the Dean of Academic Affairs that afternoon.

I went to see Dean Scarborough, and he informed me that I now held the record for a college that dated all the way back to 1781, for the lowest grade point average ever! But he had examined all of my previous academic records and said, "Fred, I *know* you can do better than this. You have great potential. I believe in you so I'm placing you on academic probation. You have one more semester to prove yourself and show us what you're really capable of. Don't let me down. If you screw up again, you're out."

Long story short, I made deans list that next semester, and the semester after that and the semester after that. I graduated with an enviable GPA. I figured out how to take care of business first (study) and still have plenty of time left over for fun.

Lesson number one: You have the innate potential to do better, to feel better and function better than you may now see at this moment in time. Someone else has faith in you that you can be a better version of yourself.

Dean Scarborough believed in me. Well, I believe in *you*. Why? Because we've seen the success of countless other patients who did not believe they could get any better... and they did.

By the way, my friend Gordy went on to graduate from Point Park College and have a successful career, but he never returned to W&J. I graduated from W&J in 1972 and went on to Emory University Dental School. I got married to my beautiful wife of forty-two years while in dental school and we had our first child while in school also.

My next story about my education has the same theme. It's again about problems I encountered with enrollment (yes, apparently lightning does strike twice) but with a different moral and lesson.

When I went to enroll for my senior year at Emory University Dental School, I was invited to visit George H. Moulton, the dean of the dental school, and speak with him. Dr. George Pryles, my advisor was there also. Together they advised me to drop out of dental school.

Mind you, this was my *senior* year. I had already successfully completed three years at Emory with a B plus academic record.

They told me that I would never make it as a dentist, that I didn't have what it takes. Even though my academic record was excellent, I was a little slow in clinic and had not completed the number of units of fillings, crowns, bridges, etc. that we should have had done by then.

However, what I did complete was excellent, and... I wasn't that far behind. I asked them whether they could force me to drop out of school and they said they could not. But they reiterated that I would never make it as a dentist and strongly advised me to take their advice and withdraw.

I told them if they could not *require* me to drop out that I was staying. Now what? They informed me that that I would not graduate with my class of 1976 and instead would be held back another half year. I agreed. So I quietly graduated in 1977 in the latter part of the year all by myself. No cap. No gown. No ceremony.

I went on to create a highly successful reconstructive practice, become a clinical instructor and regional director of one the most prestigious post-graduate dental teaching institutions in the world, spoken to and educated dentists from all over the world, been featured on the magazine covers of our profession's biggest journals, consulted with major dental manufacturers on the development of new dental products, been interviewed on NBC and CBS talk shows and spoken at our profession's biggest meetings... I could go on.

Unfortunately if I do it's going to seem like I'm bragging or trying to impress you. I'm not. Here's my point. *I went on to prove them wrong.* If I would have taken the word of naysayers, I never would have gone on to a successful career and have had the opportunity to change the lives of so many people.

Lesson number two: Don't let *anyone* tell you what you can or cannot accomplish. We place doctors in too high of esteem. Well, guess what? They're human. They make mistakes just like you and me. If someone has told you there is no cure for your pain or that's as good as it's gonna get – don't take "no" for an answer. Don't accept their words as a life sentence.

The human body has some amazing capabilities and abilities to heal. If you are still in pain or poor function – do not give up. Prove the others wrong. You have the ability to function and feel better than you currently do. I truly believe this and so should you.

You are a magnificent creation of God. Your health and power are innate – on a level of *being*. Don't give someone else the power to condemn you to a life of chronic pain.

One last dental school story. It was April 4, 1977. Dean Moulton walked into our senior class and said a Southern Airways jetliner had just crashed in New Hope, Georgia. There were a lot of fatalities. They were shipping all the bodies to the Fulton County Medical Examiner's Office. He needed four volunteers from our senior class to go down to the morgue and take dental records on the corpses to help identify the bodies.

Alas, no hands went up. No one volunteered. So he went alphabetically. Abeles. Number one.

We arrived at the Medical Examiner's office amid chaos. There were seventy-two bodies in black body bags, zippered up. They were all burned beyond recognition. Women. Children. Men in business suits. All charred completely black with their flesh burned off.

The smell was horrendous. I had worked on cadavers in dental school as we studied anatomy but this was an entirely different beast. These were all regular people like you and me who had been alive just a few short hours earlier.

Seventy-two lifeless bodies in a small space. There were arms, heads and legs that did not have an owner. I was a little scared but didn't want to show it. All four of us were disoriented and confused – what do we do? Where do we start?

Someone showed up and handed us little power saws. We had to saw open their mandible (lower jaw) to get their mouth open and then chart all their teeth, fillings and dental restorations. Since the bodies were burned beyond recognition, it was hoped that the airline would use the passenger list, try to obtain dental records from all the family dentists who had seen these passengers, match up our teeth charting and attempt to identify the bodies so they could be transported home to their respective families.

We got a sort of sick little rhythm going after cutting open about a half dozen corpses and charting them. Lots more to go. My head ached. My mind raced with a million thoughts. All these dead people and no one even knows who they are. They have families just like me. They were someone's husband, wife, father, mother, sister, brother.

My clothes were sopping wet with my sweat. Some guy joined me. He had the biggest needle and syringe I'd ever seen in my life. He plunged it straight down into their chest and extracted fluids into it.

We worked all day and well into the night. They brought us food from McDonald's. I didn't care. Who could eat? Not me. In fact, I couldn't eat for over twenty-four hours.

The vision of those seventy-two lost souls, the smell and the sadness of the group there that fatal day, stayed with me for a long time. This life event brings us to the third lesson...

Lesson number three: Life is short. Don't take anything for granted. We can be here today and gone tomorrow. As it applies to our work together in this book – don't take your health for granted. If something is not functioning properly, if something does not feel right, if you don't feel like yourself – get help. Don't accept things as they are and think you'll get around to it some time in the future.

Your health is one of the most precious things you possess. Cherish it, nourish it and protect it. It can be gone in a flash.

One last story for now and then we'll move on to the next chapter. I have two beautiful, amazing children, Jennifer and Jeffrey. Along with my wife, they are the love of my life. But both of my children have had serious, life threatening health problems at an early age.

My daughter Jennifer, had a stroke at age 31. She had to walk with a cane, had speech problems, balance problems. But she would not accept this as a life sentence. She fought her way back to a full recovery. If you met her today, you would never know the pain and dysfunction she endured for years. She would be bright, articulate and energetic. She envisioned herself healed and whole and did not stop her quest until she achieved it.

My son Jeffrey, has already had two major surgeries, one life threatening. He has requested I do not go into details here, so I will not. But understand that at a tender young age he experienced more pain and disease than anyone would want to endure.

Again, if you met him today, he is not only healthy and bright, but he would appear like someone you would see in a fitness commercial on TV. He's buff, eats well and takes great care of himself to protect his body and health.

I wish no parent to ever endure what my wife and I have gone through with our children's health crises. We've learned that our health is so fragile and must be nurtured and protected. We've learned from our beautiful children that with encouragement, faith and proper care, our bodies can heal and recover from even life threatening disease.

Lesson number four: Don't wait for a serious wake-up call to finally decide you want to feel and function better. The time is now. Take positive steps to improve your situation and don't stop until you're rehabilitated.

It's your turn to shine. It's your turn to enjoy your life pain free. It's your turn to feel alive again.

I know my connection with my patients and empathy for their condition was heightened as a result of these four experiences. It certainly is not the route I would wish for any other doctor to discover they want to spend their lives helping people get free from pain – but it certainly worked for me. This is my calling. Now you know why I wrote this book – to help people like you change your life.

Pain

LET'S START THIS chapter off with a bang. Sadly, most of what you think you know about pain is wrong. For example: most of our pain in the head and neck comes from the nerves, right? Wrong. Most of the pain originates in the muscle and connective tissue.

Ok, well how about – pain is bad. Wrong again. You better rethink your premise here. Trying to immediately mask your pain with two Advil and ignore it thereafter ... may turn out to be the worst thing you can do, even though that's what we've seen a thousand times being done on TV. Pain can be beneficial – *if heeded.*

Pain is our body's 'check engine light'. When the warning light flashes on the dashboard of our car, it's a clear signal that something is not working properly in our car and if ignored will probably get worse and continue to cause damage until we eventually have a catastrophic engine failure and the car stops running.

Well, pain serves the same function in our body. We don't have an electrical signal to turn a flashing red warning light on in the palm of our hand, but we do have a signal that travels down our nerve pathways and ends in an impulse of pain.

Just like our car, we can ignore the warning signal. Remember the old AMCO transmission commercial with the guy who said, "You can pay me now, or you can pay me later"? There was a lot of truth in that catchy phrase.

Something that mechanically is not functioning properly will slowly deteriorate until it ceases to function at all.

The same applies to our vehicle, our body. If we receive a consistent pain signal and all we do is ignore it, then there's going to be undesirable consequences in the future. If something is not functioning properly in our body and we are receiving warning signals by experiencing daily pain – we can ignore them and allow the problem to progress and worsen, or we can pay attention and seek proper help.

It's not rocket science. If we have pain, our body is telling us something is not right. Pay attention. Get it fixed! Yet what do most of us do? We try to *mask* the pain symptoms with the latest new wonder-drug pill we saw the dancing, smiling people taking on the television commercial. In essence, we not only ignore the warning light, we cut the wire under the dashboard that goes to the light so it won't flash any more!

That's pretty much what we do every time we pop some pain pills to mask the pain. We ignore our body's amazing early warning system and instead we short-circuit it with pills. Basically we cut the wire so the warning light won't flash any more.

Does that sound like a sensible approach to dealing with problems with your car? If the engine is making clicking sounds and not running properly, do you really believe by ignoring it that whatever may be malfunctioning is just going to spontaneously heal itself?

If your computer suddenly flashes a warning sign that it has a virus, do you un-install your anti-virus program so that you won't see the warning message any longer or do you attempt to delete the virus before it causes further damage to your computer?

Well then, why oh why do we act in such a stupid manner when it comes to something as precious as our own human body? If our warning system is firing off red danger signals should we continue to ignore them or deactivate the warning system? Or should we take action to identify the problem and stop it from causing further damage and deterioration to our body?

If it sounds like I'm belaboring the point here, you're correct. I have seen thousands of patients over many decades in my career and it still amazes me how many apparently highly intelligent people come into my office and tell me they have been taking pills for years to deal with their chronic pain and they know they have a problem that is getting worse. So listen up.

There's a 'disconnect' in our brain between logic and reason. We may know on a logical basis that smoking is detrimental to our health and can cause cancer - or that overeating and a poor diet can cause diabetes and heart disease. But we do it anyway.

So the same illogical thought process is in effect when dealing with our chronic pain. We may know that something is wrong and we should seek proper help to correct our malady before it causes even further damage to our system – but we don't!

Instead, incomprehensibly, we disconnect the warning light completely. Let's take some more pills and temporarily make the pain go away. Just understand that if the underlying problem that is causing the pain is not corrected, even if we mask the pain, the system will continue to deteriorate and the problem progresses and worsens.

Eventually, when enough damage has occurred, we are usually forced to seek care, but by then the degeneration may have advanced much further. Remember, "Pay me now, or pay me later."

Here's an unpleasant truth – Many of you reading this book will not get better from your headaches, migraines or TMJ dysfunction.

This statement may make some of you angry or shocked or doubt my credibility but I feel I have to share this information with you for two reasons.

First, it's simply true. We know from our many years of experience in practice that most headache and TMJ remedies out there don't work for long. We also know that the vast majority of patients who go from one doctor to another, chasing one magical cure after another in hopes it will take their pain away, fail. The medical literature is full of studies showing the lack of efficacy of many symptomatic treatment modalities.

Secondly, I am sharing this information with you and putting our potential new relationship at risk because I believe *the only real chance you have to get better is to first acknowledge this reality*. Once you admit that what I've said is in fact true, you can begin to examine why this is so.

Let's start with the most obvious reason: Trying to just mask symptoms of pain instead of identifying the root cause of symptoms is doomed to long-term failure. I'm going to repeat it. Trying to just mask symptoms of pain instead of identifying the root cause of symptoms is doomed to long-term failure.

If you can finally accept this as truth, then you can be helped.

We have the ability to choose. We can choose to live with pain and try to mask it or we can choose to identify the source of the pain and eliminate it. The choice is yours and there are consequences to each choice.

The physiology of pain is complex; however a few basic principles can take you quite far in terms of being an informed patient.

Most pain in our body comes from muscle and fascia (the connective tissue intertwined with our muscle). Knowing this one simple fact gives us a lot of power to correct the cause of pain.

The precursor to pain is inflammation. If we can reduce inflammation in our muscle and fascia, we can reduce pain. As you will discover in following chapters, our work centers on identifying the source(s) of inflammation in muscle tissue and improving the muscle's physiology and function. Happy muscles do not create pain.

I understand that 'happy' is not a scientific adjective to quantify muscle function, but I'm determined to keep this book simple and understandable for you without a lot of fancy medical jargon and long words. For now just know that when muscles are functioning properly they do not create pain.

Here's a final thought I'll leave you with: It may be impossible to find the world's best cure for pain. But sometimes the worst one is hard to miss. Stop trying to mask pain with pills.

The Many Faces of TMJ

TMJ IS AN ACRONYM for temporomandibular joint. Our lower jaw can also be called our mandible. Our skull has a large bone on the side of head called the temporal bone. Ever heard someone say they got hit in the temple? It's based on the name of the underlying bone; the temporal bone.

Where these two structures meet together is called the temporomandibular joint. It's in front of your ear. It is a hinge joint that allows our lower jaw to open and close. It's a hinge joint with a few very unique 'twists' that our other joints don't possess. If you put your fingers on your head right in front of your ear and open and close, you can feel your TMJ move.

Most joints in our body are a basic ball and socket design. The ball rotates in the socket allowing the limb to move. For example, if you bend your arm and raise your hand, your elbow joint rotates and allows your upper and lower arm to move. It's basically a rotating ball and socket joint that is functioning in your elbow.

With rare exception, most all of the joints in the human body function in a similar manner... except one. The TMJ.

The TMJ is the only joint in the human body with three unique characteristics:

First – It's the only joint in the body where the left and right joints have to work together simultaneously in perfect harmony. Every other joint in our body, we can work the right side independently and separately from the left side.

With the TMJ, both joints have to work simultaneously when we bite, chew, open/close our mouth, yawn and swallow. They are called dihedral joints, which simply means that even though both joints are working at the same time, each joint may be undergoing a slightly different movement and trajectory.

Second – It's the only true sliding, gliding joint we have in our body. When we open our mouth and our lower jaw opens, the TMJ is not undergoing a pure hinge rotation. It is simultaneously sliding down and forward as it rotates.

The 'ball' of the TMJ, which the technical name is the condyle or condylar head, not only rotates, but it slides down and forward at the same time!

The 'socket' portion of the joint, the technical name being the Glenoid Fossae, has a slope to the front of it, and the condyle just slides right down this slope as it rotates.

Third – It's the only joint in the body that has 28 teeth stuck between the opening and closing motion to complicate things and potentially mess things up.

Think about it, every other joint in our body has its position, movement and range of motion completely controlled by our muscles. The only joint that has a bunch of teeth stuck in between the opening/closing motion to complicate things, is the TMJ.

For example, when you raise your hand, your biceps contracts causing your elbow joint to rotate and voila, your arm moves. The entire movement was mediated by muscle. The position of the joint, its range of motion and the movement were all controlled by your brain sending a signal to the muscle to act upon the joint and presto, your arm moved.

Not so with your TMJ. In this case, when you close your mouth and your lower jaw comes up to meet your upper jaw (your maxilla), we've got fourteen lower teeth and fourteen upper teeth that have to mesh together.

And wherever the hills and valleys of your upper teeth and the hills and valleys of your lower teeth fit together, that's where your lower jaw aligns. It's kind of like the gears of two pieces fitting together, and wherever those gears mesh together easiest, is where they will fit.

So your 'bite' or 'bite relationship' (where your teeth all fit together) aligns your lower jaw. The position of your lower jaw is *completely* determined by where your teeth fit together. Well, part of your lower jaw, is the condyle, the 'ball' of the ball and socket in your TMJ. In essence, the lower half of the TMJ joint, the condyle (the ball) is positioned by your bite.

So basically what we're saying is this... your bite determines the alignment of your lower jaw which determines the position of the ball in the socket of your TMJ. Simply stated – the TMJ is the only joint in the human body where the position of the joint is entirely dictated by where a bunch of teeth come together.

If your bite relationship is basically compatible with where the joints should be, we can go eighty to ninety years in our body and never have a problem or even be aware of how the joints work.

However, if our bite relationship aligns our lower jaw and thereby the jaw joints in an incorrect position, too far back, too far up, twisted left, twisted right, tipped down, tipped up, etc. then all the muscles that have to support, stabilize and move the jaw become worn out from working 24/7 trying to stabilize the lower jaw and the jaw joints in a position where they shouldn't be.

And guess what? Tired, worn out, stressed muscles create pain. They create symptoms. If the joint position is incorrect, then the tendons, the ligaments and the TMJ disc all can develop problems also.

Keep in mind, the TMJ has two main moving parts – the condyle, and the disc. Let me explain...

The condyle is the 'ball' of the ball and socket. The condyle is part of our lower jaw. It moves when our jaw moves. The Glenoid Fossa is the 'socket' in our head, our skull. The socket is fixed. It doesn't move.

The good Lord, in his infinite wisdom, when he designed our joints, said we shouldn't have bone rubbing against bone. If the bones touched and rubbed, they would degenerate and become arthritic very quickly. So he put a little cushion, a little shock absorber in between the ball and the socket. It's a fibrous disc – a tough, cartilaginous piece of tissue designed to go between two bones and protect them from hitting each other and deteriorating.

The disc is the other main moving part. Both the disc and the condyle move down and forward together when we open our mouth. Remember, the TMJ is the only sliding, gliding joint in our body.

So we open our mouth, our lower jaw moves. The condyle rotates and slides down and forward. The little disc comes down and forward with it, to act as a cushion, a spacer, keeping the two bones from touching.

How does the condyle and disc move down and forward you ask? There's a muscle called the lateral pterygoid that attaches to both of them. The muscle has two heads – a top head (superior head) and a bottom head (inferior head). Yes, a two-headed muscle.

So when we open our mouth, the lateral pterygoid muscle pulls both the condyle and the disc down together as one unit. On the back side of the disc, there's a rubber band. It's called the posterior collateral ligament.

It works just like an elastic band. The more you stretch it, the more it wants to spring back to its original shape. So this posterior collateral ligament tethers the disc in place. When we open our mouth and the condyle and disc move down and forward, the ligament (think rubber band) stretches.

When we close our mouth, the condyle and disc go back and up. The ligament pulls the disc back up into its normal resting position right on top of the condyle. Pretty cool design. We've got a built in movable shock absorber that cushions and protects the two bones from touching each other and breaking down. Here's where it gets tricky...

If the condyle isn't in the right position – it's too far backwards or too far upwards – then there isn't room for the disc to sit on top of the condyle. The functional space has been reduced and the disc sits out in front of where it should be.

Again, there's a muscle pulling the disc forward when we open (the lateral pterygoid). If there's not room for the disc to rest and sit on top of the condyle, then the lateral pterygoid muscle pulls the disc forward, and *it sits in front of the condyle instead of on top of it.*

Now we open our mouth, the condyle rotates and slides down and forward. When it reaches the mal-positioned disc that's sitting out in front of where it should be, the condyle pops on the disc. That's the 'click' or 'pop' we feel when we open our mouth if our jaw is popping!

When we close our mouth, the condyle slides up and backwards and it slips back off the disc and we can feel another 'click' or 'pop'. The condyle slipped back off the disc. The disc sits out in front of the condyle. Sound complicated? It is. But hang with me here...

Some of you reading this might be asking, "Ok, the condyle is too far up or back and there's not room for the disc so it sits out in front of where it should be. But *why* is the condyle too far up or back?" Good question.

Remember we said the TMJ is the only joint in the human body where its position is dictated by where a bunch of teeth come together. So if our bite aligns our jaw too far up or too far back, then the jaw joint is too far back or too far up. *That's* why the disc is out of place and we click or pop.

We're not done yet. The clicking and popping doesn't actually create our pain. Neither does the disc, the tendons or ligaments. The pain comes from our muscles.

If our muscles that support, stabilize and move our lower jaw and TMJ joints are tired and worn out from trying to hold and stabilize our joints in a position that they're not supposed to be in (too far up, too far back) – then the muscles fatigue, wear out and create pain.

The key takeaway point: Unhappy muscles produce pain. Unhappy muscles produce symptoms.

Remember the story of the canary in the coal mine? In days gone by, miners would bring a canary in a cage into the coal mine with them. The canary would serve as an early warning system of an *unseen* danger, carbon monoxide or methane gas in the mine that could kill them. The canary would die first and serve as an early indicator to vacate the mine immediately.

The clicking and popping in the jaw, is the 'canary in the coal mine' that shouts that the jaw and TMJ are not in the right position and serious unseen problems lie ahead. If we click or pop, our jaw is too far back or too far up. Period.

The sounds in the joint are the warning sign that the joints are not where they should be. The muscles that then have to hold and try to stabilize the jaw in this incorrect position, eventually fatigue and wear out. The muscles create the pain. Got it?

But be aware – you don't *have* to click or pop to have a problem. Many people with headaches, migraines, vertigo and various other head and neck pain, *never* click or pop but still suffer from TMJ dysfunction that is the underlying cause. I know, I know – it's confusing. Want me to go on? It gets worse...

If the bite positions the jaw too far up or back and the disc sits out in front for too long, the rubber band that holds the disc in position, can stretch, become lax and lose its ability to pull the disc back to where it should be and tether it in place. Slowly over time, the posterior collateral ligament stretches further and further, becomes more and more lax and the disc migrates further and further forward, away from where it should be resting on top of the condyle. The further away the disc migrates, the more difficult it becomes to ever get the disc back in place and the worse the prognosis becomes.

Here's a simple way to tell how far away your disc is from the condyle (no MRI needed).

When you open your mouth, if you click almost immediately upon opening, before your mouth is open far at all, that means the disc is still very close to where it should be. Think about it – if the click occurred as soon as you barely opened, then the condyle did not have to rotate and slide very far before it reached the disc and popped on it. That's good! This is pretty easy to correct.

If you open your mouth about half way and then you click, that means the disc is further away, the ligament is further stretched and the condyle had to slide further down until it ever reached the disc to pop on it. Not so good. Worse prognosis.

Worst of all, you open your mouth and open almost all the way (really wide) and then you feel a click or pop – the condyle had to slide much further until it reached the disc to pop on it. The disc is much further away and the posterior collateral ligament is really fatigued and stretched. This is the worst prognosis.

And the problems are only beginning. Now we may not be able to pop back on the disc at all. If that happens, the disc now acts as a little 'roadblock' and it prevents the condyle from sliding down and further forward. When this occurs, we can't get our mouth open all the way.

The typical response is, "I woke up today and I can't get my mouth open all the way. What happened?" The disc, which is now well out of position, is preventing the normal travel of the condyle and we can't open.

Eventually, the disc degenerates and the posterior collateral ligament can be torn or perforated. We were meant to function on the tough, fibrous disc. It is designed to go eighty, ninety years between two bones and protect them without wearing out.

The ligament is basically a rubber band. It was never meant to be functioned on and it can perforate. Now there's nothing standing between the two bones (the condyle and the fossa). The disc is gone. The ligament is perforated. You know what happens next...

We say, "I used to click and pop. That stopped a while ago. And now all I hear is a grindy, gravelly, sandy sound in the joint. I can't open much and it really hurts. What is that?"

That sound is made by the condyle rubbing against the glenoid fossa (the ball against the socket). It's called crepitus. The two bones are contacting and then the bones themselves deteriorate.

Understand, this is a degenerative joint disease. Left alone, it slowly gets worse and deteriorates. First there's just some muscle dysfunction and soreness. Then there's disc dysfunction. Eventually the disc is destroyed and the ligament along with it. Then there's bone degeneration.

It's actually not that much different from degenerative joint disease in a hip or knee. If the mechanical dysfunction is ignored long enough, damage progresses and more tissue is destroyed.

So, here's a good question for you. Why does anyone decide to ignore all these obvious signs and symptoms of degeneration? Don't they understand how things progressively get worse over time? Sure they do. But they are a victim of the 'normalcy bias'.

The normalcy bias basically demonstrates that human beings tend to deny possible adverse consequences that they have never experienced before. For example, the residents of New Orleans, even though they were warned to evacuate when hurricane Katrina was approaching, never had experienced a flood of epic proportions so they did not believe it could actually happen to them.

Many people stayed home and then suffered the devastating consequences of Katrina. *They just didn't believe circumstances could become that bad since they'd never experienced anything like that before.*

Sadly, we see many patients who are victim to the normalcy bias. They just never believed that their condition could degenerate so rapidly and severely until it was too late because nothing like this had ever happened to them before.

TMJ has been called the 'Great Imposter' because so many symptoms can manifest from its dysfunction. Certainly the most obvious symptoms can be things like clicking and popping in the jaw, pain in the joint when we open, close, bite something or chew our food, grinding sounds in the joint when moved, pain around our temple or jaw, etc. Those types of symptoms are quite obvious there's a problem with the joint.

As an analogy, if our knee or hip was popping or grinding when we moved it, or had pain every time we moved it, we'd know that something mechanically was not working properly in the joint.

Yet, there are less obvious symptoms that still emanate from TMJ dysfunction, so you may not be feeling pain for the reasons you think. This category includes headaches, migraines, blocked/stuffy ears, ringing in the ears, dizziness and neck pain. Many patients have spent years chasing remedies from assorted health professionals to no avail.

Most headaches can be relieved or eliminated when the muscles of the head and neck stop producing pain. We'll talk more about specific solutions in future chapters, but for now, just know that temporomandibular joint dysfunction can go undiagnosed by many physicians and if the underlying cause of the pain is misdiagnosed, there won't be a positive outcome.

Here's a key point: *You can't cure what you don't have.*

If the problem is misdiagnosed, the solution won't be effective. This sounds so obvious and simple, yet large numbers of doctors and patients alike rush headlong into treatment, sometimes with powerful drugs and yet a correct diagnosis has not been made.

Almost everything in the human body that malfunctions has a cause and effect. Things don't happen because of random bad luck. If one is an astute enough clinician and diagnostician, the underlying cause can be determined and successfully treated.

So first get the facts. Be thorough. Think. Then treat successfully.

"Many men would rather die than think." – *Bertrand Russell.*

Headaches and Migraines

ERE ARE THE facts – According to the International Headache Foundation, forty-five million Americans suffer with chronic headaches. To put that number in perspective for you... that's more than all the sufferers of diabetes, asthma and coronary heart disease *combined*.

Hugh Jackman, Ben Affleck and Janet Jackson are all famous migraine sufferers. Headache and migraine pain can affect anyone but women are three times more likely to experience them as men.

More than half remain undiagnosed either due to misdiagnosis or failure to seek help. Living with a chronic condition can be emotionally difficult and many sufferers experience depression or anxiety as a result of their condition.

The American Migraine Prevalence and Prevention Study (AMPP) commissioned by the National Headache Foundation found that less than half of people suffering from migraines received a correct diagnosis; and among women the percentage is even lower.

Many just try to dismiss their symptoms as "just a headache" and fail to seek help. Others may be reluctant to seek help because migraines may co-exist with depression and anxiety and be afraid they would be labeled as psychologically unstable and not taken seriously.

There are no specific medical tests to diagnose migraines. Physicians make the diagnosis of migraine merely from the symptoms reported by the patient.

They're undertreated. More than half of the sufferers rely exclusively on over-the-counter pain relievers for attempted relief. Many do not use Inderal, Topamax, Imitrex, Depakote, Zomig, Relpax or Maxalt to treat their migraines because of either a bad experience with the medication, undesirable side effects from the drugs or just attempting to self treat the condition. There are two main types of migraines; with or without aura. An aura is a group of symptoms that accompany the headache including visual, sensory and cognitive changes.

Without aura – About 80 percent of migraine sufferers have a migraine without aura. The headache may last from several hours to several days, primarily felt on one side of the head with a pulsating or throbbing quality. The pain is moderate to severe in intensity and may be aggravated by routine physical activity such as walking or climbing the stairs. During the headache there may be nausea, vomiting or increased sensitivity to light or sound.

With aura – About 20 percent of migraine sufferers have a migraine with visual symptoms such as flickering lights, spots or lines or even temporary decrease in vision, or difficulty speaking. Again the headache may last from several hours to several days, primarily felt on one side of the head with a pulsating or throbbing quality. The pain is moderate to severe in intensity and may be aggravated by routine physical activity such as walking or climbing the stairs.

While a migraine may be the best known type of headache, all head pain and facial pain from headaches are not migraines.

Cluster headaches create intense often excruciating pain on one side of the head and face and may be accompanied by symptoms such as flushing , congestion or even a swollen eye. The pain is often described as stabbing or knifelike and it can radiate toward the eye or jaw. These headaches often come in clusters or packs in frequent periods over a few weeks to few months.

The headaches can last from fifteen minutes to a few hours. Unlike most headache disorders, cluster headaches are more common in men. These headaches involve the trigeminal nerve (fifth cranial nerve). Because the pain of a cluster headache is usually on one side of the head it can be misdiagnosed as a migraine. One distinguishing characteristic of a cluster headache is that it can cause a general sense of restlessness and agitation, whereas migraine sufferers feel the need to withdraw and rest in a quiet, darkened room.

The International Headache Society defines cluster headaches as five or more episodes of head pain that meet the following criteria:

Severe one-sided pain above the eye or temple area, accompanied by swelling, redness or tearing of the eye on the same side, congestion or runny nose on the same side as the facial pain, swelling or drooping of the eyelid on the same side, sweating of the face and forehead on the same side, and a sense of agitation or restlessness.

Tension headaches are the most common form of headache. Like migraines, they are more common in women than men. The pain from a tension headache can feel like a tight band encircling the top of the head or a vise squeezing the head. The pain can range from mild to severe and it differs from the migraine and cluster headache in that it is usually felt on both sides of the head and there is no nausea involved.

In some cases the entire head can feel tender or sore to the touch and pain may be felt in the back of the neck.

Most family practice physicians, internists and neurologists tend to approach headache and migraine therapy with prescription drugs. Some drugs are designed to prevent symptoms from worsening from the initial onset. Others attempt to lessen symptoms once the headache is full blown.

Unfortunately, in all cases the medications are designed to provide relief from symptoms from the headache rather than treat the root cause of the headache. Here is a list of medications commonly prescribed for headaches or migraines. Pick your poison:

Imitrex – A triptan drug delivered by nasal spray or subcutaneous injection. It's not recommended for people with certain heart problems. Side effects include flushing of skin, tightness in chest or throat, fatigue, dizziness and muscle weakness. People with a history of heart attack, stroke, angina or atherosclerosis should not take triptans as they can constrict blood vessels.

Zomig – A triptan drug delivered by nasal spray and oral form. Side effects include dizziness, dry mouth, sweating and weakness. Zomig should also be avoided by people with heart problems.

Ergotamine – This drug is available in either injectable, inhaler or sublingual form. Nausea can be a problem with this medication and can be serious if used frequently.

NSAID's – Non-opioid pain relievers such as Advil, Motrin, Aleve and Toradol are all non-steroidal anti-inflammatory drugs. Because they are non-addictive they are used very frequently for treatment of headaches and migraines. However they should be used with caution because of the significant side-effects including: edema (fluid retention), nausea, vomiting, diarrhea, constipation, heartburn, kidney and liver problems, stomach bleeding and more.

Opioid pain relievers – Drugs such as Demerol, Darvon, Oxycontin, Actiq, Stadol and others are not designed specifically for use in migraines or headaches but rather, are for general pain relief. Most are available in oral form. Overuse can cause physical dependence and increased tolerance to the drug requiring ever-increasing doses to have effect. Side effects include nausea, vomiting, memory loss, confusion, fatigue, itching and constipation. They can depress respiration and breathing so they should be used with extreme caution with other drugs at bed time or with patients with respiratory problems.

Migranal – An ergot derivative class of drugs along with Ergomar are an older class of migraine medications. Because of the high incidence of side-effects especially nausea, these drugs are only used as a last resort when other drugs are contra-indicated. Side-effects include peripheral vaso-spasm (blood vessel constriction) which can restrict arterial blood flow and tissue death.

Depakote – A drug classification of valproic acid that can help prevent future attacks. Frequent blood and liver tests are required for patients using this drug for headache or migraine therapy.

Chances are if you visit a neurologist they will perform a battery of tests to assess your motor skills and function including a mental status assessment, cranial nerve tests, motor and sensory systems, deep tendon reflexes, coordination and gait analysis. You will probably have either an MRI or CT scan.

If you visit an endocrinologist they may say you have a high or low thyroid. If you visit an allergist or ENT they may say you have sinus problems. Your cardiologist may say it's a peripheral circulation problem. What they all have in common is this…

When you ultimately leave their office, you will probably have a new prescription in your hand to treat your headache or migraine symptoms. Some drugs are to be taken daily just to try to "prevent" symptoms. Others are for when you have pain.

If you're happy with the results of the painkiller, gained significant relief, have minimal side-effects and are coping well with your headaches or migraines, then just work hand in hand with your physician to monitor the ongoing effectiveness of the drug and any effect on organ systems that may result from its prolonged usage.

Chances are if you're reading this book, you're not doing so well. If you've already tried prescription painkillers and are not pleased with the results, then stay with us and learn how you can relieve your headache or migraine safely, predictably and effectively.

Let's get to know the true enemy: Ninety percent of pain comes from the muscles.

The temporalis muscle is the major positioning muscle that moves your lower jaw upward and backward thousands of times per day. If this muscle is constantly trying to hold the mandible in a position that isn't correct, the muscle becomes fatigued and sore. Look at the position and size of the temporalis. Can you see how this large muscle can affect your headaches?

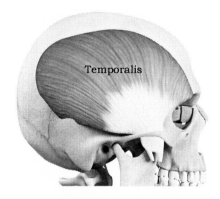

Temporalis

Please understand this: Your bite, the way your teeth fit together, dictates where the tmj/jaw joint has to go. One controls the other. Your bite controls your jaw joint position. Then the muscles have to hold it in that position.

Now, if your bite positions your lower jaw even half a millimeter further backward or upward or torqued or rotated… the muscles have to compensate and hold the jaw in the improper position dictated by where the teeth fit together. All day. Every day.

Imagine if I asked you to raise your arm and hold your arm straight out sideways. Now imagine if I asked you to hold this position for three hours. How about three days? Do you think your shoulder muscle (deltoid muscle) would be sore and painful? It would. Why?

It will be painful because the deltoid muscle that positions your shoulder will become fatigued from holding it in a position where the muscle cannot return to a state of rest. It's working overtime. Circulation will be impaired. There will be a build-up of lactic acid in the muscle that will cause pain. Lymphatic drainage will be compromised. Fatigue, soreness and pain will set in.

This is the same process that results when your temporalis muscle has to hold the lower jaw in the wrong position. I've deliberately oversimplified this process for you to understand it and maybe have a little 'aha' moment and say, "Ok, now I get it."

Yes, there are other muscles involved in headaches besides the temporalis, but the principle is the same. This is why we're able to have such a high degree of success treating headaches. Even if the original source of the headache is not muscle pain, if we can get the muscles of the head and scalp which participate and contribute to the pain more relaxed, the headaches can be reduced or eliminated.

The cause of the headache is as important as the headache itself. Get an accurate diagnosis.

It's essential to get the diagnosis right to ensure the desired treatment result. Your goal isn't to just mask the symptoms of your headache or migraine pain. You want to determine the root cause of your pain first to achieve your goals – whether they are relief of pain, reducing or eliminating previously prescribed drugs, becoming more active or just having more good days than bad days.

Many people think that headache therapy involves prescribing medications, sinus surgery, injecting Botox or following some strict dietary guidelines purported to avoid triggers and avoid the onset of pain. The truth is that you have to identify the critical elements that contribute to the pain and onset of symptoms before making any changes to your body with drugs, surgery or diet.

Two things should be jumping out at you here:

1) Most physicians haven't really made a definitive diagnosis as to what is actually *causing* your headaches versus just trying to treat symptoms.
2) Drugs don't work very well for headaches. Well medicated, by the way, doesn't mean well cared for.

So let's take a closer look at the true enemy...

Here's the real culprit – inflammation, muscles of the head and neck, forward head posture, bad bite, cervical alignment and its effect on the cranial nerves and vertebral artery. Let's have a go at these one by one.

Inflammation is the precursor to pain. Before tissue sends noxious signals through nervous pathways to the brain that are interpreted as pain... there is inflammation in that tissue. If we can reduce inflammation, we can reduce pain.

When the muscles of the head and neck are stressed to the max and fatigued from trying to support and stabilize the mandible in an incorrect position, the muscles fatigue, rest is impaired and inflammation occurs.

And remember... the discrepancy in the bite relationship doesn't have to be huge. A tenth of a millimeter in the wrong direction is enough to create a problem. We're dealing in micro-trauma here, tiny discrepancies, not macro-trauma.

If you carry your head out in front of your shoulders, you have a condition referred to as forward head posture. From a side view, your head ideally should be centered over your shoulders. In a side view, an imaginary line drawn from your ear should bisect your shoulder.

If your ear appears in front of your shoulder, then by definition, you have forward head posture. Here's the significance – the further forward you carry your head in front of your shoulders, the more stress it places upon the muscles of the head and neck that have to support your head.

Our head weighs approximately eight to ten pounds. If it is centered on our shoulders, our cervical spine can ideally support its weight. However, if our head sits in front of our shoulders it places a tremendous stress upon both the cervical vertebrae in our spine and the muscles that stabilize and support our head.

Imagine this – You have a ten pound bowling ball in your hand. You hold it right in front of your chest. It doesn't feel too heavy if you hold it there for just a moment. Now imagine you hold the bowling ball with your arms outstretched further away from your body. How does the bowling ball feel now? A lot heavier!

The further out in front of your body the ball goes, the harder it becomes to support it and the more stress it places upon your muscles. Can you imagine trying to hold the ten pound ball well out in front of your chest for a few hours? How about all day?

Even though we don't think about it, that's the same scenario that plays out day by day if we have forward head posture.

And the *reason* we have forward head posture? A bad bite.

Next, the alignment of our top three vertebrae in our neck, C1, C2 and C3 are affected by the position of our TMJ. For example, if our bite relationship positions our left TMJ slightly further back than our right TMJ, we will see the identical relationship in C1, and C2. They will be torqued, twisted to the left and match the degree of displacement in the condyles.

Said another way - the position of our jaw joints affect the position of our neck vertebrae *and...* the position of our neck vertebrae affect the position of our jaw joints. There is an inter-relationship between the two structures. One affects the other.

Keep in mind that our cranial nerves and vertebral artery have to snake through our cervical vertebrae on their way up to the brain. If there's torque in the mandible and resulting torque in the cervical vertebrae... there's torque (twisting force) exerted on the cranial nerves and vertebral artery.

It's like crimping a garden hose. The water doesn't flow through it properly. So it shouldn't come as a surprise to you that torque in our cervical vertebrae compromises the blood flow and nerve signals to our brain.

Sooner or later, you're going to realize that there's no mystery to this. As I stated, everything has a cause and effect. Find the cause. Cure the effect.

Some of you may be tired of hearing me talk about the bite relationship affecting the jaw alignment affecting the muscles affecting the nerves and creating pain. But the facts speak for themselves.

Knowing what you now know, does it come as any surprise previous attempts that didn't address these issues failed to relieve your pain? Perhaps, more importantly, now that you understand the true cause and effect of headache and migraine pain - do you still want to mask it with drugs – in essence buying a lottery ticket with your health?

The Pharmaceutical Industry:
Where there's Pain there's Profit

LAST YEAR AMERICAN pharmaceutical companies spent $3.5 billion dollars advertising drugs on TV. We then spent $325.8 billion dollars buying them. No other country even comes close. So are we the sickest country in the entire world or do we watch too much TV?

One thing is for certain. It's big business. The pharmaceutical companies spent $2.7 billion dollars last year just on lobbying. That's more than any other industry. And that's 42% more than the second highest paying industry – insurance.

So who benefits the most from all these ads? You? Big Pharma? The insurance companies?

Here's a little hint (it's one of the most important lessons in medicine): The easier it is to mask symptoms with a quick fix pill, the larger the underlying problem will eventually grow. And to keep symptoms at bay, you have to keep buying the drug.

Sound familiar? The pharmaceutical companies are banking on your *repeated use* of their products. So to figure out who gets the short end of the stick, just invert the question. Who stands to gain the most if the underlying problem is not corrected?

Answer: The pharmaceutical companies.

The public places far more value on a big budget slick TV commercial with a bunch of smiling, dancing people, flowers and pretty music designed to push their hot button for the latest wonder drug that will solve all their problems, than on the less glamorous approach of detailed diagnostics to determine what actually is wrong and fixing it.

How do we fix 'stupid'?

Even worse, we've created a nation of hypochondriacs by parading a bevy of disorders from insomnia, depression, erectile dysfunction, seasonal allergies, high cholesterol, toenail fungus, bi-polar and other mood disorders in front of consumers all day and all night on TV.

How well does all their advertising dollars work? Like the potato chip commercial says, "Bet you can't eat just one." Twenty percent of our population is now on five or more prescription drugs. Ka-ching! So many pills. So many choices. We know we can't keep taking pills forever... and yet we can't stop.

As a result of Madison Avenue's slick TV ad campaigns, the patients tell the doctors what's wrong with them and what pill they want to fix it. We're reducing doctors to order takers. It's no exaggeration to say that our medical treatment is now being influenced by television commercials propagated by big pharmaceutical companies. In essence, we are by-passing the MD. There are billions of dollars at stake here - and your health.

"Drug ads strengthen our belief in pharmaceutical drugs as the cures for all of our problems. In fact, the consequences of poor lifestyle choices cannot be undone by pills. Many advertised drugs are not only ineffective, but have serious side effects that are frequently played down and occasionally concealed by manufacturers. Thirty second TV spots that trade on emotion and celebrity contribute little to nothing of value to patient education."

- Andrew Weil MD

We've become a nation of pill takers. Got a problem? There's a pill for it. We're so easily influenced by advertising. It's bad enough that we make purchase decisions for our clothing, our liquor, our cars, our vacations and so much more by what we view on TV.

But surely not our health? I hope, as a result of reading this chapter and doing your own thinking for yourself you'll be able to spot the flaw in this cultural phenomenon that is unique to the United States. (The only other country that's stupid enough to allow direct-to-the-consumer drug advertising is New Zealand).

Stop being influenced by pharmaceutical ads on TV. Most all of these drugs have serious side effects, some life-threatening. Sometimes it's not until years later that they discover the damage a drug can do to us. I challenge you to listen to the last thirty seconds of these manipulative productions and actually pay attention to all the risks and things that can go wrong when you take these pills! It's your health and organ systems we're talking about here.

What Americans are about to learn the hard way is – there's no quick fix, no magic pill and no free lunch when it comes to medical problems. And here's one more point to consider. I saved the best for last.

Even if the new pill you saw on TV is successful in masking your symptoms and taking your pain away for a while, if the underlying medical problem goes untreated your condition worsens. All you have accomplished is to kick the can a little further down the road.

At some point, usually after things have gotten far worse, the patient is forced to seek proper medical care to address the actual cause of the problem and discover that five years worth of pills only benefited the pharmaceutical company.

Most people are not adequately informed of the potential harm to their body and organs they risk with frequent or daily use of these drugs. You can see for yourself.

The FDA (U.S. Food and Drug Administration) announced actions taken to inform the public of the dangers of all NSAIDs (non-steroidal anti-inflammatory drugs.) The actions include changes for manufacturers in the marketing of COX –2 inhibitors, as well as prescription and non-prescription (over-the-counter) NSAIDs.

After analyzing data provided from long-term studies completed *after* the release of these drugs on the market, a joint meeting of the FDA's Drug Safety and Risk Management Advisory Committee along with the National Cancer Institute and National Institute of Health concluded there is:

Increased risk of heart attack and stroke

Increased risk of liver damage, kidney failure and fluid retention

Increased risk of bleeding stomach ulcers

Increased risk of bleeding, perforation and obstruction complications from ulcers (NSAIDs are now the second major cause of ulcers)

Increased risk of damage to the lining of the upper intestine

Here are some highlights of the FDA's recent actions:

Merck has been asked to withdraw Vioxx from the market due to the connection between Vioxx and heart disease and increased heart attack

Pfizer has been asked to withdraw Bextra from the market because, "the overall risk versus benefit profile for the drug is unfavorable." Pfizer has agreed to suspend sales and marketing of Bextra in the U.S. pending further discussions with the FDA.

The FDA has asked Pfizer to include a boxed warning label with Celebrex stating an increased risk of cardiovascular events and potentially life-threatening gastrointestinal bleeding associated with its use.

The FDA has asked manufacturers of all other prescription NSAIDs to revise their labels to include the boxed warning stating an increased risk of cardiovascular events and potentially life-threatening gastrointestinal bleeding associated with their use

The FDA has asked manufacturers of all over-the-counter NSAIDs (Aleve, Advil, Motrin, Bayer, Excedrin, etc.) to revise labels to include more specific information about potential cardiovascular and gastrointestinal risks as well as a warning about potential skin reactions.

To read the entire FDA warnings and changes call 1-888-INFO-FDA.

Here's some of the medications included in the FDA warning:

- Celecoxib brand name Celebrex
- Valdecoxib brand name Bextra
- Rofecoxib brand name Vioxx
- Diclofenac brand names Cataflam, Voltaren, Arthrotec (combination with misoprostol)
- Diflunisal brand name Dolobid
- Etodolac brand names Lodine, Lodine XL
- Fenoprofen brand names Nalfon, Nalfon 200
- Flurbiprofen brand name Ansaid
- Ibuprofen brand names Motrin, Motrin IB, Motrin Migraine Pain, Advil, Advil Migraine Liqui-gels, Ibu-Tab 200, Medipren, Cap-Profen, Tab-Profen, Profen, Ibuprohm, Children's Elixsure, Vicoprofen, Combunox, Note: there are over-the-counter ibuprofen products and many OTC combinations.
- Indomethacin brand names Indocin, Indocin SR, Indo-Lemmon, Indomethegan

- Ketoprofen brand names Oruvail, Orudis, Actron, Note: there are over-the-counter ketoprofen products.
- Ketorolac brand name Toradol
- Mefenamic Acid brand name Ponstel
- Meloxicam brand name Mobic
- Nabumetone brand name Relafen
- Naproxen brand names Aleve, Naprosyn, Anaprox, Anaprox DS, EC-Naproxyn, Naprelan, Naprapac, Note: there are over-the-counter naproxen products.
- Oxaprozin brand name Daypro
- Piroxicam brand name Feldene
- Salsalate brand name Disalcid
- Sulindac brand name Clinoril
- Tolmetin brand names Tolectin, Tolectin DS, Tolectin 600

Does anyone else see a problem here? Let's review: The pharmaceutical companies developed new drugs, advertised them successfully directly to the consumer who bought them and used them. Then years later they discover the stuff is killing you or doesn't work. Only in America.

We gamble with our health and our lives with the FDA as our watchdog. You'll get better odds in Las Vegas. I would like to nominate the FDA as the least likely federal agency to protect our health. If you want to risk your life and organ systems on the latest new 'wonder drug' you see pimped out on TV, best of luck. You'll need it.

Enough lies. Big Pharma won't stop because there's too much money in it. But at least tell yourself the truth. Just face it – there's no 'magic bullet'. Even Dirty Harry used a *six*-shooter.

If I were elected President, the first act I would perform in office would be to ban these commercials for life. Just like the tobacco ads, these would be taken off TV.

Anyone can wear a white coat on television. Not everyone knows what is actually best for your health, especially if their interests are first served by selling you prescription drugs you continually have to refill. Do your homework.

The Health Profession's Big Secret Revealed

FEW PEOPLE UNDERSTAND how important getting a proper diagnosis is before proceeding with treatment. We're the 'microwave' generation. We want everything instantly. You have high cholesterol? No problem. Here's a pill for that. Take some Lipitor or Crestor.

Can't sleep? Here's some Ambien or Lunesta. Your back is hurting? Here's a quick surgical solution. Feeling depressed? No problem. Here's some Zoloft or Prozac.

We want the easy way out. We want immediate relief. We want the quick fix.

Well, you'll have no problem finding it because most of the medical profession is geared up for quick fixes. But let's revisit the examples mentioned above...

You have high cholesterol? Take the statin and your HDL/LDL decreases quickly. But there are those pesky side-effects again. Muscle weakness (which can be a sign of a life threatening reaction to the drug) and increased risk of developing cataracts. But hey, we got our cholesterol down right away. What else could I do?

How about learning about nutrition, modifying your diet (stop eating all that crap) and getting some regular exercise every week like cardio three times per week and a little strength training? Nah! Too hard! Too much effort. It would take weeks or months to make a noticeable difference in lowering my cholesterol.

Shame on you - you can do better than the quick fix pill. Why settle for the second rate solution when you have a better alternative? You only have one body, one life and one go-around.

You can't sleep? Take some sleeping pills. Never mind the side-effects, the tolerance you build up to the drug, the fogginess, memory loss, mood changes or thoughts of suicide. I want a solution to my insomnia *now!*

Going to a board certified sleep specialist MD and having a PSG (polysomnogram) sleep study done is expensive and takes more time and effort. I don't want to do all that. Then I might have to wear a CPAP (continuous positive air pressure device) or MAD (mandibular advancement device) and require follow-up titration of the device. And it costs more... Can't I just take a pill?

Our entire medical system, insurance system and pharmacy system is optimized to deliver quick-fix solutions. The average MD, when confronted with a patient who is seeking care for headaches or migraines does not make a definitive diagnosis. They just give out prescriptions to block or mediate pain.

That's the little secret I was teasing with the chapter title. You want fast? You got it. Just be careful what you wish for.

I'm not faulting the physicians. They sincerely want to help their patients. And we would be in a lot of trouble without them. But when it comes to chronic pain, they're too quick to say, "Here, try this prescription and let me know how you're doing." Then if the patient returns and states the drug isn't helping they give them another one to try. This is the all-too-common scenario.

For example, the 'diagnosis' of the condition called Fibromyalgia is basically a catch-all for so many conditions of pain. A common treatment approach includes dispensing the drugs Neurontin or Lyrica. They dull the nervous response. Translation: "We don't really know what the hell is wrong with you, so try this medication and see if it helps."

Now, I can imagine you saying to yourself, "Now, wait a minute Dr. Abeles. Aren't there instances where high cholesterol is genetic?" Or, "Improving my home and work relationships helped but I'm still depressed." Or "I had an acute injury and the pain went away shortly thereafter."

Of course, there are situations where taking medication is the proper approach. But simply defaulting to the quick-fix approach is dangerously flawed and short-sighted. My purpose here is to give you pause to consider - to see the wisdom of the long-term approach - to understand that we can't always solve a problem with the fastest, easiest approach.

I want you to have the knowledge and context to make a better, informed decision when it comes to your health - to change your values. With a little luck... maybe I get so far inside your head that I will ruin you for life when you see drug ads on TV, and against making snap decisions to utilize quick-fix solutions.

You've come to me for advice on how to end your chronic pain. Start with yourself:

· Never underestimate yourself.
· Never feel unqualified to make decisions about your health.
· Never be impressed or intimidated by authority, credentials or degrees behind a name.
· Never blindly follow advice if it doesn't make sense to you or feel right.
· Never discredit your own common sense, intuition or judgment when it comes to your own body.

Few people understand how important it is to have a proper diagnosis before beginning treatment. How can you solve a problem before you have conclusively determined what it is? So please... slow down. Ask questions. Don't underestimate the ignorance of the American public or the shortcomings of our health system. *Take responsibility for your health.*

The first thing you must do is accept the fact that you are responsible for your current situation. Before you react defensively and curse me out, read the sentence again. I didn't say you are the *cause* of your situation. I said you are responsible for it.

By taking responsibility for your current condition, you're also taking responsibility for your future. Nobody else can do this except you.

Life has a way of punishing irresponsibility. So blame Life if you want. Or blame God if you wish. But if you want to move beyond your chronic pain, blame the only person who can ever change and improve things: *you.* Make better decisions regarding your health and take action on them.

"The question isn't who's going to let me – it's who's going to stop me?" - Ayn Rand

Sooner or later most people come to their senses. Patients show up on our doorstep after they have exhausted all the quick, easy remedies and have downed a thousand different pills to no avail. My hopes are after reading this book you will be able to arrive at a lasting solution *sooner* not later.

I want you to think about how this current madness of quick-fix-pill-popping-symptom-masking might end. Perhaps more than any other doctor you might know, I'm warning that there will be serious consequences for the short-sighted decisions we've been making.

But masking symptoms with quick-fix solutions can feel so good as they're unfolding that it's easy to forget what's really happening behind the curtains to create the faux good health we're enjoying. So here's a gentle reminder. Let's take a look at the consequences of masking some symptoms and allowing the underlying condition to continue to deteriorate:

Nobody wakes up one day and says, "Wow, today I think I'd like to go get a new hip or knee or tmj." Like any part of the human body, if a system is not healthy and stable, then it's slowly and surely degenerating. Just as a hip or knee can degenerate to the point where they eventually require total replacement, so does the temporomandibular joint.

The earlier your condition falls on the continuum of degeneration, the easier it is to resolve, the better the prognosis, the less time and effort involved to recovery, the greater the stability of the tissues and the more complete the healing. The later your condition falls on the continuum of degeneration the worse the prognosis, the more time and effort involved to recovery, etc. The earlier treatment is pursued, the greater the chance for recovery.

Presented below are the facts. They're presented here not to scare you or convince you to pursue treatment. Everyone should and can make their own choices regarding their life, health and finances.

The facts are presented here to help you understand what is actually going on in your joints. The TMJ is arguably the most complex joint in the human body. It is the only joint where both the left and right joints have to function simultaneously in complete harmony. It is the only joint that does not just purely rotate. It is a gliding, sliding rotating joint. It is the only joint in the human body where the end point in the range of motion is not dictated by muscle. In the TMJ, the end point of our range of motion is dictated by when and where the teeth come together with our bite. If our bite forces the joint into a less than optimal position, problems can develop.

Temporomandibular joint disease starts innocently enough with only muscle incoordination (dyskenesia) caused by muscle fatigue or atrophy. As the disease progresses, actual morphologic physical changes to the hard tissues (the condyle, the fossa and the disk) and the soft tissues (the tendons, the ligaments and muscles) occur.

Clicks or pops indicate that the disk in the joint is displaced forward out of place. The click is the sound made when the condyle temporarily pops back on the displaced disk. The second click upon closing, if felt at all, is the sound made by the condyle popping back off the disk again.

Throughout the entire continuum of dysfunction, the muscles that affect the positioning of the TMJ, our jaw, our bite and whole upper body posture are majorly involved in the process. If the bite and joint are not working together properly, the muscles will be sore and fatigued causing pain. To put it simply:

Muscles are muscles. Hold your jaw in the wrong position for an hour, and it's like chewing gum non-stop for twelve hours. Either way, you end up with tired, sore muscles. Your muscles don't care. They'll just produce pain if you abuse them.

Headaches, facial pain, neck pain, shoulder pain and limited range of motion can all be the result of muscle dysfunction. As stated previously, over 90% of the pain and dysfunction starts and ends with the muscles.

You can probably make an educated guess of where you fall on this continuum. We can determine precisely where you are and what your likely prognosis is.

1. Muscle soreness and tenderness. There is occasional pain around the joint when opening or chewing.

2. Occasional clicks or pops in the joint when opening. The sooner the click occurs upon opening, the better the prognosis for recapturing the displaced disk. Clicks are classified into three categories; early opening click, mid opening click and late opening click.

The early opening click occurs early in the opening cycle. In other words you feel a click almost as soon as you open your mouth. This means the condyle is not displaced far posteriorly and the disk is still close by in front of the condyle. Since the distance traveled by the condyle to get back on the disk isn't far, the click occurs quickly when we open.

The mid opening click occurs about half way between when your mouth is fully closed versus fully open. The condyle is displaced further posteriorly and the disc is further away in front, therefore it takes more time for the condyle to reach the disk and get back on it. This click has a more guarded prognosis for recapturing the disk (getting you back on your disk permanently), stabilization and healing.

The late opening click occurs late in the opening cycle. In other words your mouth is pretty wide open before you feel the click. The condyle is retruded significantly posteriorly and the disk is displaced far in front as the ligament that tethers the disk back in place is now more damaged, stretched and fatigued. Therefore it takes even more time for the condyle to reach the displaced disk and get back on it when opening. This click has a poor prognosis for complete recapture, stabilization and healing.

3. Intermittent clicking and popping. The sounds occur more frequently. There may now be multiple sounds when opening or closing the jaw. The jaw may begin to deviate to one side when opening slowly. It does not open perfectly straight up and down any more.

4. First episode of closed lock. You try to open your mouth normally but you are unable to open as wide as normal. What has happened is the condyle was unable to get back up on the disk at all, so the disk acts as a 'roadblock' preventing the condyle from sliding down and forward, so you can't open fully.

5. Intermittent closed lock. Two or three episodes have now occurred, possibly over an extended period of time, where you were unable to open your mouth fully. Each time it eventually went away. Unfortunately all the while the disk is further deforming, the ligament that tethers the disk in place is fatiguing or tearing and the degeneration is progressing.

6. Completely locked out, anteriorly displaced disk. The disk is now permanently displaced in front of the condyle and the condyle is unable to get back on the disk at all. At this point the clicking or popping ceases. The click was the sound made by the condyle when it rode back onto the disk. Now that the disk is too far displaced and deformed, the condyle cannot get back onto it, hence there is no more click or pop.

At this point you are functioning on the posterior collateral ligament and retro-discal tissues.

7. Degeneration and thinning of the retro-discal tissue. Unfortunately these tissues were not designed to be functioned on by the condyle, so they degenerate and perforate quickly.

8. Perforation of the retro-discal tissue, the posterior collateral ligament and/or the lateral collateral ligament leading to further instability in the joint.

9. Crepitis. Clicking and popping has ceased. The disk is stuck out front. The ligament that was acting as a shock absorber in the absence of the actual disk, is now perforated, so for the first time there is now bone rubbing on bone. The condyle and the fossa (the ball and socket) are rubbing against each other. There's no cushion or shock absorber in between them any more.

The sound made by the bone rubbing on bone is a sandy, gravelly, crackling, grinding type of sound. This is called crepitis.

10. Accelerated degeneration of the condyle and fossa. The bones of the TMJ ball and socket joint break down from the pressure and compression. There's a loss of vertical height in the joint. The muscles that position the joint shorten and atrophy.

11. Compensation begins in the contra-lateral joint (the other TMJ joint) due to the dysfunction in the original joint.

12. The degenerative process repeats in the other joint.

13. Bi-lateral closed lock. Severe degeneration in both joints. Unable to function, open or chew properly.

During this entire process, the muscles are compensating for the incorrect position of the condyle/fossa and they fatigue and spasm causing many varied pain symptoms.

The main point for you to understand is that TMJ dysfunction is a degenerative disease that slowly but surely progresses from normal function to muscle in-coordination, to disc movement, to disc displacement, to early joint degeneration, to advanced joint degeneration.

Regardless of where you choose to receive treatment, get help. Don't ignore symptoms. They will progressively worsen over time and the underlying structures will degenerate. Don't mask symptoms. Don't take the quick-fix route. You will regret your decision at some point in your life.

What they call 'symptomatic relief' only gets you so far. After that, it's pain again from the muscles and joints until you mask it again. Bring that approach seven days a week for 10 years and you actually *might* wake up one day and be looking for a new joint.

Answer these three questions to assess if a particular treatment modality is an effective option or a potentially damaging waste of your time, effort and money:

1) Is it sustainable? For example, can you continue to take drugs such as anti-inflammatories and pain killers over a long period of time or will they cause damage to your liver, kidneys, heart or stomach? Can you take them indefinitely?

Will chiropractic adjustments or massage therapy create lasting structural change or do they have to repeated indefinitely for any results?

Botox injections need to be repeated every three months. For how long will you choose to get injections? Six months? Six years? What happens when you stop?

If you can't sustain the therapy over the long run and make it part of your life, then any results will be temporary and potentially destructive.

2) Is it addressing symptoms or the actual root cause? In other words, is it curative or merely palliative? Drugs, Botox, massage therapy, NTI devices, dental night guards and chiropractic adjustments all deal with symptoms and attempt to relieve them.

If the therapy is providing symptomatic relief only, at what point will you grow tired of the effort to diminish symptoms and lose your motivation to continue?

3) Is it forcing your body to change or allowing your body to change by making it healthier? Or stated in a simpler way, does it work against Mother Nature or with her? For example, surgery forces your body to change. Sinus surgery for headaches, arthrocentesis for tmj pain, Eustachian tube balloon dilation for blocked ears, even injection of Botox for migraines create change but at a cost of increased risk of complications, relapse or failed surgical results.

What treatment solutions have you already tried and failed with, that did not meet these three criteria? There's a saying, "Just because you can - doesn't mean you should."

Remember the blockbuster movie, Jurassic Park? A billionaire investor used genetic technology to bring extinct dinosaurs back to life. He created a theme park where all could see his marvelous, extinct prehistoric beasts in the present.

One of the characters in the movie was the scientist Dr. Ian Malcolm, played by actor Jeff Goldblum. Dr. Malcolm made the point that everyone got excited by what they could do, but they never stopped to ask the question if they should do it.

That's a question anyone considering treatment for TMJ pain or dysfunction, headaches and assorted related problems should ask themselves. Even if you can – temporarily – mask your symptoms with many of these treatment approaches, should you?

Even if you can – temporarily – kick the can a little further down the road with a quick-fix approach to reduce your symptoms, should you? It turns out in Jurassic Park there was one small consequence they hadn't considered. The beasts kept insisting on eating the tourists.

While many people are busily racing to try the latest wonder drug their doctor gave them, or night guard their family dentist mentioned, they can be potentially sacrificing the longevity of their joints, muscles, tendons and ligaments while the true underlying problem remains undiagnosed, untreated and continues to degenerate causing further deterioration.

We have become an instant gratification society increasingly focused on shorter-, shorter-, and shorter- term results with patients and doctors alike willing to mask symptoms today at certain serious risk and damage to long-term health.

The allure of the quick-fix approach may satisfy some temporarily. But be prepared to endlessly chase and always need the 'next great thing' when securing a lasting solution fails. You have to weigh that carefully.

If you intend to have healthy joints, muscles, tendons and ligaments for your entire life then leaving a mess for the next doctor five years from now may not be the best strategy for you. You can mask symptoms. *But just because you can, should you?*

The choices you make today have a great influence on how well your body heals, how well you will function in the future and how much pain you will have for years to come.

Ask yourself this: What is 'totally unacceptable' to you? I observe that very few people have extreme clarity. Most people make excuses. They compromise. They settle. They hope it will improve. They give it one more chance – fifty times. They draw a line in the sand and then back up and draw another and another.

You have to be *frightened*, not just worried that your body isn't working properly. *Decisive*, not just wishful. Do not accept masking pain as acceptable. Little problems, given enough time and leeway, grow into bigger problems.

As Ross Perot once said (and I've embellished it here): If there's snake loose in the building, don't form a snake committee, don't do research about snakes, don't try hiding from it. Get a big stick and kill the damn thing.

Treatment Options

ECIDING WHERE TO pursue treatment can be a daunting proposition. Depending on how much research you choose to do before selecting treatment, the process can be completely overwhelming.

The amount of information at our fingertips is nothing short of amazing today. Is it a blessing or a curse? Our parents didn't have to contend with the degree of information overload we experience. The internet has created a plethora of information available to us with a simple mouse click.

But how do we separate the facts and good advice from the bad advice? Unfortunately, along with the advent of freely available information and opinions comes the fact that anyone with a website or blog can post information and write about any subject they choose, whether they are qualified to do so or not. It is incumbent upon us to discern the accurate information from the erroneous. Your health hangs in the balance.

So here, in no particular order, are the health professionals you can choose to provide treatment for your headaches, migraines, TMJ dysfunction, vertigo, stuffy ears and other related maladies:

· Family MD
· ENT

· Dentist
· TMJ specialist
· Neurologist
· Orthopedic specialist
· Orthodontist
· Oral surgeon
· Endocrinologist
· Chiropractor
· Physical therapist
· Massage therapist
· Acupuncturist
· Healers and other alternative medicine practitioners

Let's go through these treatment options from A – Z and discuss the pros and cons of each one. We'll discuss the fine print, the risks of each treatment option to help you get this right.

1) The family MD. They are a logical first stop if you're experiencing headaches or migraines. Many times they may be the 'gatekeeper' for referrals to other specialists on your medical plan. Unfortunately, their usual approach to pain management may be the dispensing of prescription drugs to try to relieve your pain.

They most probably will not even attempt to treat TMJ dysfunction, as this does not really fall well within their domain. The bad news, which will repeat itself with the other medical specialists, is that your condition may become misdiagnosed. As I mentioned earlier, you can't cure what you don't have.

Be careful that an accurate diagnosis has been made after proper due diligence and testing, not just a quick assessment that results in being told that you have 'migraines' based merely upon the number of episodes you have per month or you have an 'ear infection' because you are dizzy or your ears feel blocked.

Either of these quick diagnoses may result in a prescription for antibiotic and steroid containing ear drops for the 'ear infection' or strong analgesics for the 'migraines'. You get the idea. Just be cautious that you don't walk out the door after a five minute doctor's visit with a few prescriptions in hand. If that was the case, your chances of long term success are minimal.

2) The ENT. This of course, is a physician who limits their practice to the treatment of diseases of the ear, nose and throat. Depending on what you are suffering with and seeking care for, they can be the best choice and extremely helpful or a poor choice. Let's explore both scenarios...

First let's look at some of the problems with which an ENT can be an excellent alternative.

Dizziness. There are many causes of vertigo, but one of the most common causes is benign paroxysmal positional vertigo, mercifully abbreviated BPPV. It can cause symptoms of dizziness and nausea. It is caused by little crystals that are in our otolith organ of our inner ear becoming dislodged and floating around in our endolymph (the viscous fluid in our little semicircular canals that is a vital and integral part of our entire balance organ.)

A change in head position, such as lying down or turning our head left or right can trigger an onset of symptoms. So head position is involved in the onset of BPPV. There is a simple test your ENT can perform to determine if someone has BPPV.

It's called the Dix-Hallpike test. The patient's head is quickly reclined and turned to one side. If someone has BPPV, their eyes will dart in a motion called nystagmus. It's a clear, telltale sign/symptom that someone has BPPV.

The good news... it's easily treated and cured. The Epley maneuver is a procedure that repositions the little crystals back (canalith repositioning procedure) where they should be and voila, the vertigo is gone. It's kind of like physical therapy for dizziness. It has a very high success rate.

So a logical starting point for treatment if you suffer from vertigo would be an ENT. They can screen you for BPPV and determine if that is the cause. If so, be certain your ENT does what is called 'vestibular rehabilitation' on a regular basis. If they do, you're in good hands. If not, find the best group in your community that specializes in vestibular rehabilitation.

Vertigo, in its most common form, BPPV, has an excellent prognosis.

Next up - sleep disturbances. Breathing disturbances during sleep can cause many serious, even life-threatening problems. Many times, if someone has sleep disordered breathing, the airway is partially obstructed, preventing proper breathing. This results in reduced oxygen saturation in our bloodstream.

One name given to the problem is obstructive sleep apnea, or OSA. By definition, a true obstructive apnea results in our cessation of breathing for a period of least ten seconds per event. An individual with severe obstructive sleep apnea might stop breathing for ten seconds *thirty to forty times per hour!*

A common sign of OSA is someone who ceases breathing for several seconds and then makes gasping sounds as they resume breathing. Here's the hard facts: 80% of loud snorers have obstructive sleep apnea *and most don't know it!* The vast majority of people with OSA are still undiagnosed.

Here comes the scary part. This is a partial list of diseases closely associated with obstructive sleep apnea:
· Diabetes
· Heart disease
· Myocardial infarction (heart attack)
· Stroke

· Hypertension (high blood pressure)

· Impotence

· Enuresis (adult bed-wetting)

· GERD (gastroesopophageal reflux disease)

How about some statistics to get your attention here...

· People with OSA are three times more likely to be involved in a car accident

· 50% of all snorers have OSA

· To complicate things further, 50% of all people with OSA don't snore

· 75% of people with temporomandibular joint dysfunction have signs that suggest sleep disordered breathing

· A narrow maxillary arch (your upper arch of teeth) is 90% predictive of OSA

· A retruded chin is 70% predictive of OSA

· If the lateral border of your tongue is scalloped, it's 70% predictive of OSA

I'm not done yet, in fact I'm just warming up. Stay with me – this is important.

· The average lifespan for people with untreated obstructive sleep apnea is 55 years of age. In essence, it reduces lifespan by an average of 20 years!

· 17% – 20% of Americans have OSA and 90% are undiagnosed

· It's more prevalent than diabetes or asthma

· It raises blood pressure

· It increases risk for atrial fibrillation

· It increases the risk for stroke 8x. (twice as much as diabetes or high blood pressure does)

· It increases the risk of heart attack 23x. That's 3x more than the risk from smoking or high blood pressure

· It increases the risk of congestive heart failure

· 1/3 of all patients with coronary artery disease have OSA

· 15% of OSA patients have diabetes compared to only 3% in the general population

· It decreases blood flow to the brain

· 65% - 80% of all stroke victims have sleep apnea

· It impairs concentration and memory

· Imaging the brain shows changes similar to Alzheimers

· It can cause teeth grinding and clenching

· It can increase depression

· OSA increases with age, weight gain and respiratory depressing medications

Here's a little tidbit that should alarm you. 76% of physicians who are not sleep specialists do not screen for OSA

· There is no pill you can take for OSA

· People on chronic opiate meds for pain or who create multi-drug cocktails to enhance sleep have an extremely high prevalence of sleep apnea

· Over 172,000 dosing issues wound up in the emergency room last year because of insomnia (so grandma might not have gone so peacefully in her sleep after all – she might have choked to death)

· One of the common treatment modalities for OSA is a CPAP machine (continuous positive air pressure) yet 60% - 70% of CPAP users abandon its use

Had enough? Ok. I think I've made my point.

This is serious business. Sleep apnea can kill you or turn you into a stroke victim or heart attack victim. If you or your spouse/significant other have signs or symptoms – get checked!

Here's where an ENT can help. If they are also a board certified sleep specialist, then they definitely can perform a polysomnogram (PSG) on you. This is a sleep study where they look at your respiration, oxygen saturation, neurological levels of sleep and many other factors.

One of the common metrics of the sleep study is called the AHI. That stands for apnea/hypopnea index. It's basically a measurement of how many times per hour you either stop breathing for ten seconds or more (a true apnea) or have compromised breathing (hypopnea) per hour.

Based on your AHI index and other metrics, the sleep physician will decide if:

a) You have obstructive sleep apnea

b) It's bad enough to require CPAP

If they determine you have OSA and need a CPAP, then wear it! Listen to them. This is your health and life we're discussing here. Do you want your grandkids to say, "I wish grandma were still with us!" Don't miss out on life events with your loved ones. Don't shorten your lifespan. If you need a CPAP then wear it.

Here's the rub... unfortunately even the board certified ENT sleep specialist can miss something occasionally. If your AHI was not high enough to trigger their threshold for recommending a CPAP, then they may say you're ok.

But there are other levels of sleep disordered breathing that can cause serious problems without being a bonafide obstructive apnea. If you don't have a high AHI index, yet you are not getting the proper amount of oxygen saturation in your blood, you can wake up with 'morning headaches'. They are caused by a higher level of CO_2 building up in the blood and too little oxygen.

We also have what is called the RDI, or respiratory disturbance index. Even if we don't completely cease breathing, our breathing can be compromised and impeded resulting in UARS, upper airway resistance syndrome. Think of this as a problem one notch below obstructive apnea, but still capable of causing symptoms and problems.

So be sure your ENT has screened you for all of these potential problems. Be aware – if your physician says you have a problem but it's not severe enough to require a CPAP, there are other alternatives. A good one is a mandibular advancement device, or MAD. This is a dental appliance that can be constructed by your dentist.

The CPAP opens up the airway with positive air pressure. It mainly works laterally. In other words, its primary advantage is helping to open up your airway from side to side. A mandibular advancement device on the other hand, helps open the airway more in a front to back dimension. It works front to back.

In fact the two devices work well together in tandem. When an individual wears a MAD, the physicians can reduce the amount of positive air pressure required by the CPAP since the dental device is also opening the airway. The result – the patient is more comfortable… and compliant.

Just be careful. Most people don't realize that a lot of what ENT's do is – *surgery*. They can recommend a UPPP or uvulo palato pharyngo plasty, sinus surgery, turbinate reduction and various other surgical procedures. Be certain this is what you need before 'going under the knife'.

Don't get me wrong… ENT's can do a lot of wonderful things for patients, but TMJ dysfunction and headaches – in my opinion, not so much.

Next up… your family dentist. Depending upon their educational background, training and experience, the advice you receive can vary greatly.

If you complain of headaches, migraines or TMJ pain to your dentist, the most common response will be to make a 'night guard' and to "see if it helps".

A night guard is designed to prevent you from grinding your teeth together at night. People who grind their teeth during their sleep can do serious damage to their teeth by wearing down the enamel over time. Once the enamel is ground off the process accelerates and worsens.

Your whole tooth is not made of enamel. It's only on the outer millimeter or so of the tooth. The inner part of the tooth is a material called dentin. It's much softer and more porous. Once the enamel is gone on the biting surface, the dentin wears away much faster so the whole process gets worse and worse.

So the night guard is designed to slow down this destructive process. The thinking goes like this: It's better to wear down and trash a few hundred dollar piece of plastic every few years and replace it, then to continue to damage the teeth themselves. So at least for eight hours out of every twenty-four, you can't do any damage. But here's the problem...

It's not designed or capable of treating or correcting TMJ pain or its related problems such as clicking, jaw popping, headaches, migraines, facial pain, ear pain, dizziness, ringing in the ears, neck pain, etc. It doesn't correct the relationship of the lower jaw to the upper jaw. It doesn't correct the bad bite.

So a night guard is to prevent grinding at night. That's it. It's not for treating complex pain or functional issues of the head and neck. It won't work.

Or they recommend an NTI type device. They merely take a mould of the upper and lower teeth and send a prescription to a dental laboratory asking them to make an NTI. That's all that's necessary.

So the NTI is very popular because it requires no advanced study and training to utilize it. The average general or cosmetic dentist has little interest in treating complex pain and TMJ functional issues of the head and neck. That's not what they deal with on a regular basis, but they still want to try to help their patients and not have to refer them out to a TMJ specialist. It's quick and cheap to fabricate.

That's all fine except the NTI, if worn for an extended period of time, can cause an 'open bite.' That's when our back teeth hit together and the front ones are wide apart and don't touch at all. The NTI is acceptable as a 'quick-fix' however there are better 'quick fixes' in our opinion and it can help for a few days or weeks because it prevents the teeth from coming together. It helps to temporarily shut down the action of the masseter and pterygoid muscles that may be contributing to the pain. If you have one, do not wear it for an extended period of time, such as months. It can eventually open up your bite and will not permanently cure your TMJ pain and problem.

Ask your dentist how many years of advanced post-graduate study they've invested specifically in the treatment of TMJ, head and neck anatomy, physiology, TMJ therapy, TMJ pain management, bite analysis for TMJ and where they received their training. Most general dentists choose to focus their expertise in other areas of practice.

It's better to seek care with someone who specializes in TMJ related problems, who has advanced training and experience in treating TMJ disorders and the host of related problems it spawns. Unfortunately, the field narrows quickly if you look closely.

The vast majority of our profession just does not treat advanced, complex TMJ problems on a daily basis. It's not their "thing." Just please be careful and discerning in your selection.

If you go to your family dentist for help with your TMJ or headaches, another option they may suggest is called, 'equilibration'. Simply put, equilibration is re-contouring the biting surfaces of your teeth. Remember, we said the TMJ is the only joint in the body whose position is dictated by where a bunch of teeth come together. So on the surface, equilibration might seem like a logical treatment option.

Here's the problem with equilibration... 95% of the cases seen and treated for TMJ dysfunction or headaches have a discrepancy in the position of the condyles (ball) in the fossa (socket) that is far larger than merely grinding a tiny bit on the existing teeth will ever correct. Besides, in almost all cases, the condyle is compressed also.

In other words, *more* space is needed between the teeth to decompress the condyles. Taking away tooth structure by grinding and removing more tooth structure is a step in the wrong direction.

Lastly, your family dentist may suggest making you some sort of bite splint to reposition your jaw and change your bite. First, ask them to clarify if what they are referring to as a bite splint is in fact a night guard that they plan for you to wear just at night when going to sleep. The drawbacks of a night guard have already been discussed.

On the other hand, if they propose to fabricate a functional appliance that is worn during the day, you have many things to consider before consenting to the treatment. There are many dentists whose training and philosophy of treatment are based upon the premise that finding a stable, reproducible position for the condyles, where they are fully seated in the fossa, in a position that can be repeated and reproduced is the target position for your jaw and bite relationship. I advise to proceed with caution...

Be careful with any practitioner who wants to manipulate your jaw in any manner to find their bite position for you. Anyone who pushes on your jaw, holds your jaw or manipulates your jaw in any way whatsoever, is arbitrarily selecting a bite relationship for you that may not work, may not be comfortable and may not remotely solve your problems.

For example, if I took your arm and flexed it up behind your back, and pushed it up as far as it can go, I may find a terminal hinge position for your shoulder joint that is reproducible. However, I humbly suggest that the position will not be comfortable or physiologically correct.

In contrast, the proper position will be in a range where the muscles are able to function with maximum strength in complete comfort. Remember, 90% of our pain comes from muscle. If we get the muscles functioning and feeling better, we can reduce or eliminate the pain.

Let me share a little story with you here. I'll start with a confession.

I wasn't always a trusted expert on the treatment of TMJ and headaches. I have humble beginnings as do most people. In 1987 I spent a week in Palm Springs with a doctor who at the time, was considered a renowned TMJ expert, Dr. Harold Gelb. That week was my first serious foray into the niche of treating TMJ.

I studied with other experts and soon I found myself treating our patients in Atlanta for these problems. Of course, I did my very best for our patients and we had some successes to be sure. But I was approaching headache and TMJ treatment from the same manner as every other dentist:

1) Give the patient a night guard, NTI or a basic appliance
2) Give the patient some muscle relaxers
3) Hope for the best
4) If it got worse, give them some pain pills
5) If it still didn't help, refer them to an oral surgeon for a surgical consult or a neurologist for more pills

We helped some people but there were a lot we didn't. I was using the same traditional old-school approach to treatment that had always been done – and still is. Just not by us. Ok, so I'm not perfect. Who is? At least I'm being up front with you and telling you my tale of ineptitude and woe. Most try to hide their failures.

So now what? I had two choices as I saw it:

1) Abandon treating TMJ and headache patients and try something else.

2) Figure it out and actually *help* those patients in pain.

I heard about this dentist out in Las Vegas, Dr. William Dickerson, with a provocative, new cutting edge approach to treating people with TMJ, facial pain, migraines, vertigo and tinnitus. He had a teaching institute called the Las Vegas Institute for Advanced Dental Studies.

Here's the thing... they were getting amazing results for their patients! So I enrolled in the Institute, went through all of their programs and became so knowledgeable and committed to this treatment approach, that a few years later they invited me to be on the faculty as a Clinical Instructor and their Regional Director.

Today, dentists from all over the world travel to LVI to study this effective treatment approach. I've been privileged to teach there now for over fourteen years.

I stayed with it until I figured it out. I spent untold thousands of hours in study and tens of thousands of dollars in tuition for my education. But now we're so certain of our results that we offer an unconditional money-back guarantee. Our treatment regimen is unique and highly effective. Our results speak for themselves.

Ok, enough about me. Let's move on.

Next, on our list of choices for you is a TMJ specialist. This will usually be a dentist who has limited their practice to focus on the treatment of disorders of the head and neck. If you have found the right doctor, this will be treatment that they render every day in their practice, not just occasionally. Inquire about their training and background. How long have they been providing specialized care? How many patients have they treated with TMJ disorders and headaches? What specifically is their approach to treatment? What is their success ratio?

If they talk to you about muscle function, jaw position and your jaw joints – if they utilize splint therapy, cold laser and ultrasound – if they say that surgery is usually a last resort – if they make a definitive diagnosis before suggesting therapy... you're getting warm. We'll go into more detail in the next chapter about this approach to treatment.

You can see a neurologist. When we have migraines or headaches, a neurologist is a logical choice to seek help from. Most patients will not seek a neurologist's help for TMJ joint dysfunction, rightfully so. They are typically extremely thorough from an examination standpoint. You may have multiple diagnostic tests including imaging by MRI, tomography or CT scan.

The caution comes from the fact that despite all the thorough tests and being given a diagnosis, you very well may leave their office with a bunch of prescriptions. If this is their solution for your headaches or migraines then you already know my opinion. If you don't, re-read Chapter Four.

The other treatment solution that your neurologist may suggest for you is to inject Botox. Botox originally gained popularity from its ability to smooth out wrinkles on the face by relaxing the underlying muscle tissue wherever it is injected.

Over time, and with research, they discovered that not only will Botox relax muscle tissue to temporarily improve aesthetic concerns such as wrinkling, but that it can also be injected to relax muscles of the head and neck that cause headaches and migraines.

Here's a few facts related to the use of Botox for headaches and migraines:

Federal health authorities have approved Botox injections for the treatment of chronic migraines in adults. The Food and Drug Administration recommended that Botox be injected approximately every three months around the head and neck to dull headache symptoms.

The drug is made by Allergan, Inc., of Irvine, California. The two company-funded studies submitted to the FDA involved 1,384 adults from 122 study sites in Europe and North America. They found that after six months, patients who got the drug experienced fewer days of migraine than they had before the studies started.

"The benefits are modest when you look at the overall results," says Dr. Elizabeth W. Loder, associate professor of neurology at Harvard Medical School and the chief of the division of headaches in the Department of Neurology at the Brigham and Women's Hospital in Boston.

"But, of course, within those results, there are always patients who do much better than the average and there are patients who don't have any benefit," she said.

The FDA stated the most common adverse reactions reported by patients being treated with Botox were neck pain and headache. Approximately one percent of patients on the drug found that their migraines worsened to the point they had to be hospitalized, but it was generally well-tolerated.

The drug labeling warns that the effects of the botulinum toxin may spread beyond where it is injected, causing symptoms that may include life-threatening difficulties swallowing and breathing.

The actual treatment requires doctors administer a total of 155 units to each migraine patient in 31 injections into muscles of the head and neck. The treatment is then repeated at three month intervals.

Allergan recently settled a Justice Department investigation into its marketing practices related to uses of Botox by paying $375 million and pleading guilty to a misdemeanor misbranding charge. The company also paid $225 million to resolve civil claims the Justice Department asserted under the civil False Claims Act.

So now let me ask you a question.

How much sense does it make to you for someone to go to the doctor every three months for migraine treatment and have 31 injections of the botulinum toxin put into their muscles to temporarily freeze them for three months to feel better? Does that seem like a good long-term treatment plan for migraine relief to you?

If the MD's want to help by prescribing painkillers to dull pain, or inject Botox to reduce muscle pain, doesn't it make more sense to find the actual cause of the muscle pain and spasm and relax the muscles permanently by correcting the imbalance between the maxillae and mandible that caused the muscle pain in the first place?

How about using a little common sense? Before you try the next wonder drug quick-fix cure for your problem, ask yourself, is it likely to turn out well over the long term (5 years) by doing something because it's easy. That 'wonder drug' might just cause you problems.

Next up... orthodontists. Most orthodontists do not treat disorders of the head and neck such as TMJ dysfunction and headaches. However, a select few do.

Let's get back to the basics that we discussed previously. If the pain is caused by the muscles.and the muscles are not functioning properly due to supporting the jaw and its jaw joints in an improper position... then tell me which should come first:

1) Finding the correct physiological position for the jaw, joints and muscles?
OR

2) Moving teeth around?

You guessed it. First and foremost, determine the proper functional position for the jaw and jaw joints where the muscles function best, are relaxed and do not create pain. Then and only then - consider moving the teeth to match this position, to be congruent with it.

Reverse the order at your own peril. If you start moving teeth around first without determining the proper position for the mandible, condyles and muscles, tell me how you plan to arrive at the correct physiologic position?

If you planned to drive from Atlanta to Seattle – would you just start driving without a specific map of the most direct route to get to your destination? Or would you have your final destination locked and loaded in your GPS?

Same here. Don't start moving teeth until you know *where* you need to move them *to.*

In summary, orthodontics can play an integral role in your final plan of treatment, but as the saying goes, "Timing is everything." Get the physiology correct first. Then move teeth to match, if appropriate. Got it?

Oral surgeons. Like the name implies, they do surgery. Not a good fix for migraines or headaches, obviously. It's basically a last resort for joints. There are many surgical procedures for the TMJ, such as arthrocentesis, arthroscopy, joint resection, disc retention, condylectomy, coronoid process reduction and others.

Here's the problem. (I may be beginning to sound like a broken record but I'm ok with that. As my old high school teacher said, "repetition, repetition, repetition". It's how we learn.) If the underlying position of the joints is incorrect because our bite relationship is incorrectly locating our jaw in the wrong place, then even if we have surgery on the joints, the improper bite relationship persists and continues to damage the joints, the tendons, the ligaments, the disc and the muscles.

That's why we see so many patients that have had previous surgery, say they felt a little better for a while and then relapse back into pain. My goal here is to make you better informed about the cause and effect of pain of the head and neck than 99% of all other consumers, so you can be more knowledgeable and make proper decisions regarding your own health.

Although many people want might you to think you cannot play any role in your rehabilitation, and rather you should just blindly defer to their advice and judgment, I want you to be able to think for yourself and understand the basic principles at work here. Pain has a cause and effect. Treat the underlying cause and the pain goes away.

Next up... chiropractors. Chiropractic manipulation has been successfully performed for many people. There are many different chiropractic philosophies and techniques of manipulation. The best technique for the head and neck is what is called Atlas Orthogonal Chiropractic.

It is noticeably different from other conventional chiropractic techniques in that it is so gentle, the patient may not even know they have had a manipulation done. The primary purpose is to correct any misalignment of the Atlas in our cervical spine.

The Atlas, or C1 as it is also called, is the topmost vertebrae in our spinal column. It is in contact with the occipital bone which is the flat bone at the base of our skull. The Atlas is named after the Greek Mythology God, Atlas, who purportedly supported the entire world on its head.

The Atlas, along with the Axis, or C2 are responsible for a wide range of motion of our head and neck. If the Atlas is misaligned, it can contribute to a host of problems. This is the main goal of the chiropractic adjustment, to realign the Atlas.

This is all fine and good except for one little detail. The condyles directly affect the position of the Atlas. There is a clear inter-relationship between the two structures.

Let me try to give you an example. Let's say that your bite relationship positioned your left condyle slightly further back than your right condyle. Again, remember the position of our temporomandibular joints is dictated by where our teeth come together which aligns the lower jaw.

So let's say your left condyle is further back than your right one. Well, guess what? Your Atlas will be torqued to the left also; and to the same degree of rotation as the misplaced condyle.

The inter-relationship of the condyles and the Atlas is profound. If a chiropractor adjusts C1, the Atlas and ignores the left and right condyle, guess what happens? The adjustment helps temporarily, but will be undone quickly by the constant input from the condyles.

Atlas Orthogonal chiropractic can help. It can be beneficial if there is a cervical component to your pain. However, used solely by itself, if the occlusal (bite) relationship/connection is ignored, the effects of the manipulation will be only temporary in nature.

Next up... physical therapy and massage therapy. Although different modalities, they share a common thread in working to improve muscle function, range of motion, reducing trigger points, and reducing pain.

Physical therapy goes further, teaching a patient proper body mechanics, strengthening exercises designed to stabilize the joint and utilizing other methods to reduce inflammation and promote healing to injured tissue such as iontophoresis, ultrasound, heat, dry needling, cold laser and others.

Both treatment modalities can definitely help reduce pain and symptoms, but hopefully by now you have a basic understanding that I hope I have imparted to you. *If they do not alter or correct the fundamental underlying functional problem* then their solution can only be palliative, temporary in nature.

Acupuncture, which has its origins in Eastern medicine, places small needles in our muscles to reduce trigger points in the muscle. Similar to dry needling which a physical therapist might perform, acupuncture can be effective in temporarily reducing pain, however it shares the same limitations as massage and physical therapy.

Lastly, we have a large assortment of healers and alternative medicine therapies and techniques too numerous to mention here. Again, I would advise caution and performing due diligence before consenting to treatment or medicines that have not undergone proper scrutiny.

I have more confidence in a health professional who has had many years of peer reviewed advanced training from an accredited institution versus an individual who had no barriers to entry and might have been a car salesman (I have nothing against car salesmen) six months ago. If it sounds too good to be true, it probably is. So please exercise some restraint and caution.

So, what's the point of all the information in this chapter? Well, my goal was to allow you to now understand the principles behind the cause and effect of pain in the head and neck. If there is a functional problem, it requires a functional solution. If the head and neck are mechanically distorted in any manner, then the muscles that have to support and stabilize that distortion will create pain. It's vital you understand this concept.

If you ignore this fact, you will be vulnerable to any and all quick-fix treatments proposed and will continue to be disappointed with your treatment results.

Consider this - there is no such thing as teaching. There is only learning. So only keep reading this book if you're ready to think about what I'm saying and reconsider much of what you've been taught about what will heal your pain.

I can't tell you what is causing your pain or dysfunction without seeing you. But I can tell you this with absolute certainty: If you ignore the underlying cause of your pain and merely pursue treatment to mitigate symptoms... you will not get better. *This is the most important information I can possibly give you.*

You need to realize that most treatment remedies will fail. You need to understand why they fail and how they fail. Don't allow your emotions to overtake your reason. Just because you want to believe something does not make it true.

So bolt the door, turn off your phone, listen up and pay attention: Patients fail to get better because they don't have the most basic tools to understand why they are in pain - they don't know how to evaluate treatment options. And they fail because they allow the underlying problem to continue to deteriorate unabated.

I truly hope you'll take this chapter to heart. I hope you'll look back on the treatment mistakes you've made in the past and think about why they happened. It wasn't bad luck. Find a way to become better informed and you'll be on your way to becoming pain free.

Getting it Right

I N THE LAST chapter, we spoke about lots of treatment alternatives available to you and discussed the pros and cons of each. I've tried to distill the critical thinking required to make the proper decisions and empower you to be able to make those decisions.

Now it's time to focus even further and talk about how to select the best doctor and treatment solution for you.

There's only two questions that count:

1) Is the treatment addressing the underlying cause, not symptoms?
2) Is the treatment focused on the muscles?

You know by now, you better be able to decisively answer, "YES" to both of these questions. I call this 'unrecognized simplicities'. There may be a plethora of treatment options out there, but once you know what to look for, the field narrows very quickly. And you didn't need a medical degree to understand it. In selecting your doctor, you'll want to know about:

· Their standard of care

· Their credentials and expertise

· The right tests to have taken

· The right treatment to have performed

Let's take a look at each of these criteria.

First up, their standard of care. This is the one that is most difficult to discern. We have to pull back the curtain a little. What does the office look like? Is it modern and up to date? Do they have state-of-the-art technology? Is the office spotless? Do they respect your schedule and time? Do they answer all of your questions completely? Do they communicate well and explain everything in understandable terms? Are their fees congruent with the services provided? (In this world we get what we pay for. Low fees usually equate with a lower standard of care) Does the doctor and team spend significant time with you or are you just another 'number'?

Secondly, what are their credentials? Where has the doctor received advanced training? Not just the regular degree, but where did they spend their time in post-graduate training? How much? A few weekend courses or hundreds/thousands of hours? How many cases like yours have they treated successfully? Do they teach? Are they on the faculty of a prestigious teaching organization?

We're looking for the cream of the crop here, the best of the best. What have they accomplished in their career to distinguish themselves from their peers? How qualified are they to have you entrust them with your health and well-being?

Third... what tests will they perform? The best way I can explain this to you is to share what we do in our practice. We focus on muscle function. We use technology that measures muscle activity with computerized EMG's, while we simultaneously track the jaw in 3D to one tenth of a millimeter in accuracy. We can conclusively determine the optimal position where the muscles of the head and neck are truly most relaxed and most functional. The muscle EMG's serve as a good proxy for how the entire system is functioning.

We can then combine these two data points – where the muscles are 'happiest' and where the lower jaw and jaw joints are with precision and determine the exact position in space where the bite relationship, lower jaw, jaw joints, muscles, tendons, ligaments, and disc are all functioning at their best.

We can then take a bite relationship that captures and preserves that relationship so it can be reproduced later if desired. We evaluate the velocity and trajectory of the mandible in function, we utilize joint vibration analysis to analyze the sounds the joints and disc make if they are malfunctioning and view the precise position at which the malfunction occurs again on a computer.

We utilize a special low frequency TENS to relax the muscles of the head and neck, to improve circulation, oxygen, glucose and ATP/adenosine triphosphate (all the good stuff we need in our muscles to function properly) and simultaneously remove lactic acid and other toxic waste products from the muscle. In essence, we improve the physiology of the muscles of the head and neck so that we can determine precisely where they would like to position the mandible, where they function best, where they are most relaxed. *Happy muscles create no pain.*

I would have to write an entire book to explain exactly what we do during diagnosis and treatment. Mercifully, I won't do that to you. Instead, I'm merely hitting the high points as a brief overview. But what I want you to take away from this is:

There are a *lot* of diagnostic tests that are necessary to uncover human physiology – to determine what's working and what isn't – what needs fixing and what doesn't. In our office this high tech battery of tests takes about four hours to complete. Yes, there's also a lot of hands-on palpation, examination of range of motion, posture, gait, pain index and more.

The point is, if you're in the right practice with the right doctor, they better be spending some significant time with you and have the ability to evaluate the function of your muscles objectively. No 'subjective opinions' allowed. We need science, data and facts to base a thorough diagnosis and treatment plan on.

The Litmus Test: If you're in the right doctor's office, they'll be more focused on the physiology of your muscles than anything else.

We have a lot of patients who fly in from across the United States and even other countries who come to see us. I don't say this to impress you. I say this for you to realize how *difficult* it is for people to find someone who can actually help them! It isn't so easy.

You'll need to be discerning. You'll need to know what to look for in your doctor and your necessary treatment. And as I already mentioned, the best way I can teach you to know what to look for is to actually share with you what we do in our practice, how we go about our diagnostic and treatment process.

Getting back to the right tests, we also have to have proper images of the temporomaqndibular joints. This will allow us to see the position and condition of the joints.

The images can be captured in several ways:

1) MRI – magnetic resonance imaging

2) CBCT scan – cone beam computed tomography
3) Corrected tomograms – a computerized xray

MRI's are typically taken in a reclining position. The problem is that when we lie down on our back, our jaw falls backward also and we do not get an accurate picture of the normal position of the condyle in the fossa of the TMJ. Then the image gets interpreted by a radiologist.

Radiologists are talented physicians who specialize in imaging; however, they are not TMJ experts. They are not into the tiny nuances that we are. So the average radiologist might say an image looks fine because there is no gross degeneration whereas we are into finer details.

For these two reasons, an MRI is not the first choice for imaging. On the other hand, the corrected tomograms and CBCT both can reproduce an accurate image of the anatomy of the temporomandibular joint and consequently both can be used to analyze the condition and position of the joints.

For example, if we were to look at an image of the left TMJ and we see that the condyle was too far upward in the fossa, then we would also know that the functional space that should exist between the top of the condyle and the bottom of the fossa has been violated or compromised.

If the functional space is too small, there is no room for the disc to occupy the space on top of the condyle, so instead it sits out in front of it, pulled forward by the lateral pterygoid muscle.

So even though we cannot image the disc with a CBCT scan or corrected tomogram, if the functional space between the top of the condyle and the bottom of the fossa is too small, then we know by default, there is not adequate room for the disc to function in there and instead it sits out in front of where it should be.

The same situation exists if we see the condyle is too far backward. Again, the disc sits out in front of where it should be. And the muscles that then have to support and stabilize the joint work overtime trying to maintain a less than optimal position. So the muscles fatigue, stress out and produce pain.

See, this isn't that hard to diagnose! Proper images, proper scans of the mandibular position, proper scans of the muscle activity and voila ... we can start to put together the pieces of the puzzle of what is causing the pain and dysfunction.

Certainly there is more that we look at, far more scans of function plus evaluation of posture, head position, neck, shoulder and jaw range of motion, balance, gait, coordination, muscle palpation, relationship to the HIP Plane, velocity of motion and much, much more.

But the point is – we can take a detailed look at how the muscles of the head and neck are functioning and start to determine what is working, what isn't working, what needs fixing and what doesn't need fixing.

There's a cause and effect to everything. We do not have pain for no apparent reason or because of bad luck. If we are an astute enough diagnostician and clinician, we can make an accurate diagnosis.

Then and only then can we begin to formulate a treatment plan, a plan for therapy and rehabilitation.

Ok. It's time to start discussing treatment solutions. If we determine that a patient's bite relationship is positioning the lower jaw and jaw joints in the incorrect position and the muscles are creating symptoms – what do we do to correct the situation? What do we do to eliminate the pain and dysfunction?

By now, it should be apparent to you that if the lower jaw is in the incorrect position and the muscles are creating pain, then we need to place the jaw back in the proper physiological position so the muscles can relax and stop producing pain. Sounds simple enough. Let's go into detail on how we do this.

First, during the physiological, neuromuscular work-up appointment, we have the patient on a special TENS machine for at least an hour, usually longer. This is not TENS like a physician's office or physical therapist might use. Those TENS units are designed to temporarily reduce pain by sending a competing signal to the brain so the brain won't 'pay as much attention' to the injured area.

It functions on the Gow Gates theory of pain transmission. For example, did you ever bang your elbow or knee and then start rubbing the area right after you hit it? Well, this is the Gow Gates theory at work. We are sending competing afferent signals to the brain from the rubbing of our skin adjacent to the site of injury. The brain perceives both signals and our pain is lessened albeit only slightly. That is *not* what we are doing here.

The TENS we utilize sends an ultra low frequency signal to the muscles of the head and neck. There is a mild pulse every one and a half seconds. This electrical stimulation of the fifth and seventh cranial nerves produces an involuntary contraction and then relaxation of the muscles of the head and neck that are involved in the positioning and movement of the mandible.

Over the course of an hour of TENS, the muscles become markedly relaxed. Think of it as kind of a wonderful muscle massage, but in actuality it is far more than that.

The TENS actually improves muscle physiology. It provides the pathway for increased circulation and oxygen to the muscle. It provides the pathway for increased glucose and ATP (adenosine triphosphate) to the muscle. In other words, it potentiates the uptake of all the good nutrients that improve muscle function.

At the same time, it potentiates the removal of harmful waste toxins that build up in the muscle such as lactic acid.

Did you ever exert so hard that your muscles burned while you were exerting? That's the lactic acid in the muscle creating that pain.

So the TENS allows the muscles to achieve their proper, optimal resting length, improve physiology and allow the muscles of the head and neck to become truly relaxed.

We're not finished here yet. After the patient has been TENSing for an hour, the TENS pulse temporarily short circuits the muscle memory of where we habitually close our teeth together. Stay with me...

Remember we said that our bite relationship determines the alignment of our lower jaw and also the TMJ (temporomandibular joints). If our bite is positioning our jaw and joints in the incorrect position, then the muscles have to go along for the ride and try to accommodate/adapt to that position.

Again, the teeth determine where the jaw and jaw joints go, the muscles have to adapt to that position. As we now know, when the muscles are no longer adapting or coping with the incorrect position, they get fatigued, worn out and start to produce pain.

So our precious little TENS unit can temporarily relax the muscles *and* temporarily short circuit the ingrained muscle memory of where we automatically and unconsciously close our jaw.

Instead, after an hour of TENS, we can close our jaw on the true, correct trajectory where the muscles would actually like to position the lower jaw if the teeth didn't get in the way and mess everything up.

Stated another way – our lower jaw can now close up and down where the muscles are most relaxed and are 'happy'. We can find this envelope of motion, this path of movement where the muscles, tendons, ligaments, disc and joints all work together in perfect harmony and peace.

Now the muscles are not fighting where the teeth (our bite) positioned the jaw. They don't have just accommodate and go along for the ride. Instead, we started with the muscles. We determined where is this ideal physiological trajectory in space where the muscles, given their own druthers, would like to position the lower jaw and jaw joints?

Can you start to see the incredible power of this approach? We can actually determine precisely where the muscles are most relaxed, working best and would like to position the jaw. If we allow the lower jaw to function in this position, we have happy muscles and happy muscles do not create pain.

Although we could get an acceptable result by merely using the TENS to determine the proper trajectory for the lower jaw and joints, this is not how we actually do this in our office. While the patient is TENSing we are simultaneously tracking the position of the jaw in 3D on a computer and simultaneously looking at the functional state of the muscles of the head and neck in real time.

There's no estimation or guesswork involved. We can unquestionably determine where the muscles are most relaxed. We are reading EMGs of the muscles on our computer. When we find the best, most optimal position for the lower jaw and jaw joints – where the muscles are most relaxed – we can capture that position with a simple bite registration.

We squirt a soft material over the tops of the lower teeth and merely have a the patient close together until they are at the optimal position where the muscles are most relaxed and the joints, discs, etc. are all in their best position.

The soft bite registration material hardens over a minute or so. Then we can remove the bite registration and send it to the laboratory along with models of the patient's upper and lower teeth.

Now the lab can mount the models in the absolutely identical position we determined was best for the patient. They put the little hardened bite registration material between the upper and lower models and now they have duplicated the exact position we saw in the mouth where the patient's muscles were most functional and relaxed.

Before the models and bite registration are sent to the dental laboratory, we measure the distance between the gumline of the upper and lower teeth in three separate locations on the models. These measurements are accurate to one tenth of a millimeter, recorded and given to the laboratory.

The laboratory is then responsible for creating an orthotic that precisely duplicates this bite relationship and must have the identical measurements, again accurate to one tenth of a millimeter. In other words, there is a tracking system in place to ensure that the appliance the lab creates is absolutely spot on identical to the bite relationship we gave them.

Now we can have the patient back, deliver the lower appliance and know that it allows the patient to close, chew, function in the identical position we determined previously that is ideal for the patient.

The appliance is clear, plastic, removable and virtually invisible. It is worn all the time. Over the course of a few months, with regular return visits to balance the appliance to their muscles, it allows the patient, for the first time, to function with their jaw and jaw joints in the proper position where the musculature of the head and neck are most relaxed.

When this is accomplished, the body can do what it is innately programmed to do. Heal. Once the joints are decompressed, once the muscles are in a functional position where they are not stressed and fatigued, the pain and dysfunction can be eliminated or dramatically reduced.

All follow up visits have an hour of TENS to relax the musculature and then balance the appliance to that ideal position. Over the course of a few months of therapy, the muscles propriocept and learn the new, improved position of the bite. After just a few weeks, the patient can now bite automatically in the new, proper position. The old, pathologic bite is unlearned and the new physiologic bite is ingrained into the muscle's memory.

When the muscles no longer have to compensate for a pathologic bite, no longer have to cope with an incorrect alignment of the lower jaw and jaw joints, then the entire system, including the muscles can heal.

Actual morphological changes can occur to the bone, the disc and the muscles. It's truly amazing how our body can heal once an insult is removed that was preventing it from doing so.

There is a lot more to the therapy than I can outline for you here. Let is suffice to say that in addition to the actual orthotic therapy, there is also physical therapy, exercises to do at home and home care devices – all designed to improve muscle function and promote healing.

After a few months of therapy, when the symptoms have markedly diminished or been eliminated, the patient will have another decision to make. We refer to this as Phase II therapy. They can:

· Continue to wear the orthotic, knowing that it will periodically need to be resurfaced in order to maintain the proper bite position. Just like a roadway wears down from continual usage and needs to be resurfaced and maintained, so does the orthotic.

· Choose to wear a new Phase II orthotic that is more robust and longer lasting. We cannot use this type of orthotic during the initial phase of therapy because we need an appliance that we can add to or subtract from to balance the bite at each and every visit if necessary. This Phase II orthotic is less adjustable. However, once the proper position has already been determined, tested and proven over the proceeding months, it is now appropriate, if the patient selects this option, to make a longer lasting, more robust appliance.

· Choose orthodontics. Now that the patient has been successfully wearing the appliance and symptoms have been abated, they can choose to move their teeth to a similar position that is compatible with the proper position for the jaw, joints and muscles. When the orthodontics has been completed, the patient will no longer need to wear the orthotic. Now their teeth, bite relationship, jaw position are all in sync, in harmony and they can get on with their life without pain or the need for the orthotic.

· Choose to rebuild their teeth to the new, proper physiologic bite position with the use of porcelain crowns and veneers. Some patients have a lot of old, defective dentistry that they would like replaced, and/or do not like the appearance of their teeth. Full mouth reconstruction, building all the new dental restorations to the exact same bite position as they function in their orthotic, is a viable option for those who choose to do this.

Regardless of all the Phase II options, I do not want you to become confused. Here's the bottom line: Focus on what works. If the muscles create our pain – focus on the muscles. Despite the new wonder drugs we see pimped out on TV all the time, let me remind you of a timeless lesson:

Sticking with the basics works.

As I've written over and over, if the muscles are creating the pain, just focus on getting the muscles right. It may seem boring compared to all the new bioengineered drugs that are purported to be the 'next big thing', but it's unlikely a new drug or technology will render our approach obsolete. And arguing that muscles don't create your pain is like arguing that the earth is flat or gravity doesn't work. It clearly defies the facts and evidence.

You'll be hard-pressed to find a more consistent method for reducing pain and improving function then focusing on creating 'happy muscles'. I can't say it enough - the basics work.

The Intangibles

WHEN OUR BODY and mind are assaulted with constant pain, it's easy to surrender to it and give up all hope of being whole again. We can give in to fear and allow it to control our life and our every decision.

We read that the number one killer of lives is heart disease or cancer. I disagree. The number one killer of lives is fear. Fear can kill our dreams. Fear can paralyze our actions. It can immobilize us and make us play it safe avoiding any risk.

Yet we have to reach out with both arms to the risk of living a full, healthy life and count doubt and darkness as the cost of knowing the truth.

If you truly desire to move beyond your headaches, your migraines, your chronic pain despite all the failures that bring you here now, then know this – fear and pessimism are acquired. They are learned. They can be unlearned. They are not our natural state.

We were not put on this earth to go around being afraid. Our natural state is one of love, freedom, hope and joy.

Realize that your fears are all created by you in your mind. You can also rid yourself of these fears if you choose. All that is required is a little faith and a little courage.

If you're afraid – feel the fear and do it anyway. As Eleanor Roosevelt once said, "You must do the thing you think you cannot do."

In my many decades of practice, I have met and treated numerous patients from all walks of life and all backgrounds. But I have found a commonality in all of them.

The patients who were successful at moving forward with treatment and ultimately going on to a better life were *not* the people who were afraid of failing at the treatment result. But rather, they were the people who were *more afraid* of what their life would be *if they did nothing about it.*

As the old saying goes, a definition of lunacy is doing the same thing over and over again but expecting a different result. Do you really believe there's a pill, injection or manipulation that is going to take away all of your pain forever?

I guess in some ways I'm speaking to you here about more than your chronic pain. I'm speaking to you about your entire life. If I could crawl inside the head of my patients and the doctors and team members I have had the privilege to speak to over the years, if I could change just one thing, if I could tweak just one little screw inside their head... it would be the one that's creating all the fear and doubt they are filled with and make it go away.

Fear and doubt can hold you back from the life you dreamed about and imagined when you were young. I'm here to tell you that you still can have the life you want. Just have a little faith! Have some courage. Take some positive action. Your time is now!

You've got to get whole again – the way you were before this all started. It's hard enough as is to create success in our career and relationships. But to try to do it from a position of ill health and pain is far more difficult.

You'll have less chance of success if your body is sick. You'll have less chance of success if you're worn out from pain or you're filled with fear that's paralyzed you from taking new positive action.

As I see it, you basically have two choices:

1) Take some risks. Try some new things. Have some faith and courage to make your life better in any and all ways you desire.

2) Play it safe. Keep doing exactly what you already have been doing. Accept life just as it is. Don't change a thing for fear you might fail. Those are your choices. Which side will you be on?

What matters now: The choice you make. The action you take. We're impressed with people we see that perform courageous acts. Our heroes in the movies. Our soldiers fighting on enemy soil to keep us safe. A fireman going back into a raging inferno to save a small child.

Why are we so inspired by them? Because deep down, in our soul, we *are* them. We're all divinely human and cut from the same stock.

The world is waiting for the better version of you. The version that is fearless and pain free.

Let me share another personal story with you. I graduated from Emory University Dental School in 1977. I graduated with all the same hopes, dreams and aspirations as everyone else did. I had this dream, this vision of a beautiful, successful dental practice and doing all this beautiful dentistry on wonderful, appreciative patients.

Well, six years later, nothing could be further from the truth. I was miserable, unhappy and disillusioned. Dentistry was all hard work, no fun and not very rewarding. I felt I'd made a grievous error in choosing the career of dentistry.

I could have continued on, being afraid to take any risks or to change anything. After all, I had just invested eight years of my life and thousands of dollars in getting my education and doctorate degree.

But I decided life is too short to persist in career in which I was not happy. The good Lord had blessed me with another talent. I was an accomplished classical and jazz pianist. Music had always been a huge part of my life and my passion. I gave my first music recital at age five for my parents' PTA association in school. I had been performing ever since.

I had my first band in junior high school, 'The Stratolites'. Cool name (at the time). The front of my drummer's bass drum had The Stratolites logo on it. We thought we were hot stuff. We played for all the high school dances including the senior prom at Altoona High School. We played at the Park Hills and Blairmont country clubs in my home town. We were little kids, but our music was sophisticated enough to play for the 'grownups'.

I had performed all through college. I put together a jazz trio - piano, bass and drums. We played local clubs in my college town. We played for various other colleges. I gave a jazz concert for the Pittsburgh Music and Arts Festival. I appeared with Jerry Lewis and Vic Damone. At my own college, Washington and Jefferson, we performed every year for Homecoming with a special concert called the 'Fifth Quarter'. It was big bash after the homecoming football game for all the faculty and alumni.

Even in dental school, when I came down to Atlanta, I put together another jazz trio. We had a free publication in Atlanta called, 'Creative Loafing' that was very popular. It's still going strong to this day. It had a classified section. I ran an ad looking for a top-flight jazz bass player and drummer. This was in the early '70s and many of the jazz greats in Atlanta were just arriving and getting going then. My timing was perfect.

I hooked up with some of the absolute finest, consummate jazz musicians on the planet and we started performing together here in Atlanta. To this day, forty some years later we are still fast friends. They all stayed in their career as professional musicians. My bass player, Neil Starkey, is a living legend. He has performed with virtually every jazz great you could think of. Whenever I have a charity event or gig, they still rally and perform with me just like in the old days.

Ok, back to the point I was trying to make. So here I was in 1983. Six years into private practice and I was miserable. Now what? I had a wife and daughter who were depending on me. I was a dentist. I had studied for years to get the degree. Surely I couldn't walk away from it, could I? But if I continued on, I would continue to be miserable...

I decided life is too short to persist in a career I didn't enjoy. So in 1983, I left the profession completely. A beautiful new luxury hotel was opening in Atlanta. It was called the Waverly Hotel. It was brand new, big and gorgeous. I went to the hotel and interviewed and auditioned. They hired me as their musical director and performer.

There was a beautiful new Yamaha concert series grand piano in the enormous open atrium lobby and I performed there every day. I worked with their sales and catering teams and they kept me booked solid performing at corporate events.

I went to the largest talent agency in Atlanta at the time, Ray Bloch Productions, and they signed me to a contract. And I very quickly found myself engulfed in a brand new career – music. I got to play for numerous Hollywood celebrities, be a guest artist with the sixty-six piece Atlanta Pops Symphony Orchestra. I wrote the entire musical score for the two pieces I performed. I met people I never would have had an opportunity to meet otherwise.

All these events happened because I took a big risk. I didn't follow the crowd. I didn't play it safe. I didn't avoid making waves. I wasn't happy and I decided to risk everything I had worked for to try to improve my situation.

That's the takeaway here. *You*... have to take some risks in your life. *You*... cannot go around living your life in fear. *You*... cannot be afraid to fail. You only get one shot at this to the best of my knowledge. Make it count. Make your life the very best it can be – what you dreamed of.

If your body is not working right... get off your butt and do something about it. If your relationships or career are not working right... get off your butt and do something about it. Don't let fear hold you back.

I was more afraid of what my life would become if I *didn't* take a risk and change it up. It's ok to have your back against the wall. Sometimes that's a good place to start from because if nothing else, you're motivated! You have to be more afraid of what you will miss out on if you do nothing than being afraid of trying to change.

Back to my music story. So here I am performing as a professional entertainer in Atlanta. I was making a nice living, supporting Rhona and Jennifer. Then in 1985, the Waverly got a new general manager by the name of John Labruzzo. He was a fantastic leader. Well, one day in a conversation with John, he asked me, "Fred, what did you do before you were here at the Waverly?"

Well, I wasn't going to lie to him. You see, I never told anyone I was a dentist when I started at the Waverly. They just knew me as Fred, the musician. So I told him, "Believe it or not, I'm a dentist!"

John was so taken back by the fact that I was a dentist and a performer, that he went to the local NBC television affiliate, '11 Alive' and spoke to them about me. They decided they wanted to do a feature story about me on television. Well, never underestimate the power of the media. Within days I had scores of people coming up to me – the employees of the Waverly Hotel, saying, "Fred, I had no idea you were a dentist! I need my teeth cleaned. I need a crown!"

So I did the only logical thing I could think to do. I hooked up a small air compressor and drill to the piano in the lobby. (Just kidding). No, I went directly across the street from the hotel and found a dentist, Mike Lefkove, and asked if I could share his office one day per week. After I put the gun down he said, "Yes". (Just kidding again). But he consented, so on Friday afternoons I started treating the employees of the Waverly Hotel as patients.

Well, one day a week led to two. Two days a week led to three. And soon we were so busy and running out of room sharing space in Dr. Lefkove's office. We were at a crossroads. I was working full time as a professional entertainer and three days a week as a dentist.

Something had to give. I did some soul searching. I realized I had always had this dream, this vision of a beautiful, successful dental practice and I had never achieved it. I decided to give it one more try.

So in 1987 I opened the doors to my own new dental office. I took with me my core group of patients from the Waverly Hotel. We sent out Val Pak type coupons for $35 cleaning and checkups and we quickly got very busy. We routinely saw fifty to seventy-five new patients a month.

I performed all aspects of dentistry. Cleanings, kids, crowns, amalgams, extractions – you name it, we did it. We worked six days per work including two evenings. I still worked at the Waverly as a pianist. I would check my last patient of the day getting their teeth cleaned with my hygienist, with my tuxedo on! My practice ended at 5 PM. I was due at the Waverly at 5 PM. The hotel gave me a little wiggle room time-wise. But it was always fun to check my last dental patient in a tux.

Let's flash forward a few decades so I don't bore you to tears with the rest of my journey.

Over the many years that passed since those early days in practice I changed the scope of the practice dramatically through an incredible amount of study and training. I stopped doing any procedures I didn't enjoy. I decided it is more important for patients to come to you for who you are, what you do and what you stand for – not because you're a name on their insurance plan's list.

We're not for everybody. We have a specialized niche. We're expensive. But by golly, I'm doing what I love, what I'm passionate about. I have fun and fulfillment. You can too!

What's the point of this little story? *At so many points in my life I had a decision to make. I could maintain the status quo and keep going on as is. I could be afraid of change, afraid of failure. Or I could take a risk for something better.*

My life has unfolded the way it has, I have gone down the paths I have because I never was willing to accept the status quo, to follow the crowd, to just fit in and do what was expected of me.

The decisions I made, the actions I took created my life and all the incredible people and events that have been part of it. This is what I hope for you. Make the big decisions. Make the tough decisions. Take some risks. Take action.

Ask the right questions. Don't ask, "How much can I stand? How much pain can I put up with?"

Instead ask, "How good can I stand it?"

Well, how good *can* you stand it? How would you like your life *ideally* to be? Make *this* your starting point. Make *this* your North Star that guides your decisions and actions. You can accomplish far more than you may currently believe is practical or feasible – if you have faith in yourself and lose the fear that's holding you back.

What else do you want to create in your life that you have not yet experienced? Here are a few more questions to ask yourself:

"If I were today the person whom I hope to become... what would I do in this situation?"

"If the qualities of my life are not substantially better two years from today, how will I then feel?"

"So, what should I be doing *right now*, to ensure I will feel great about the qualities of my life in the future?"

Here's one of my favorite quotes. It comes from the book, 'Moby Dick' by Herman Melville:

"For as this appalling ocean surrounds the verdant land, so in the soul of man there lives an insular Tahiti, full of peace and joy, but encompassed by all the horrors of the half-lived life."

My hope for you is that some day, when you look back on your life, you will not have regrets for all the things you wanted to do and dreamed of doing, but did not even try to accomplish because of some imagined fear.

Be bold. Be courageous. Take some risks. Live a little. You'll be amazed at what you can accomplish.

I basically have only a few hours with you while you read this book. I not only want to change what you do, but how you think. I want to change how you think about pills.

I want to change how you think about quick-fix solutions. I want to change how you think about what you're afraid of.

So answer these questions as they relate to your pain and your life in general:

· What is my deepest fear?
· How has fear lowered the quality of my life experience?
· Who created my fear?
· How would my life be different if I did not give in to my fears?
· What is my negative thinking costing me in my life?
· Am I willing to exchange the fear in my life ... for faith? Right now?

Here's a little exercise that will only take you a few moments to do. *Please*, put your book down and go grab a piece of paper and a pen.

Just as you can strengthen your muscles with exercise, you can develop and strengthen your courage and faith to ask for what you want in your life.

As it relates to your health and your life, write down three things that you want and are willing to ask for:

_____
_____
_____
_____

Describe a current problem in your life that exists because of your fear:

_____
_____

I promise that I will:

"Faith is like radar that sees through the fog – the reality of things at a distance that the human eye cannot see."

– Corrie ten Boom

"Have faith in yourself and the universe. Have faith that if you do the right things for the right reasons, it will turn out well. Have faith that all things are possible."

– Fred Abeles

Come to the edge, he said.
They said, We are afraid.
Come to the edge, he said.
They came.
He pushed them ... and they flew.

– Guillaume Apollinaire

Case Study

OVER THE COURSE of my career we have treated untold thousands of patients. When dealing specifically with chronic pain patients the one thing that sticks out as most notable is how many of these patients had received care from previous health care professionals without a thorough work-up and definitive diagnosis being completed before commencing treatment.

One patient, a young lady in her twenties, had been under the care of an oral surgeon for nine months for treatment of her TMJ pain. The surgeon had made a splint for her to wear and had adjusted it repeatedly over the nine month period.

He had given her medication to manage her pain, which had grown progressively worse. He finally informed her that it was just going to take another six months for her to improve, for her pain to reduce and to be patient with the process.

She came to our practice in tears, in severe pain and desperate for even a little relief. During our examination it became quickly apparent to my assistant of thirteen years and me that her symptoms were not consistent with those of temporomandibular joint dysfunction.

We immediately conferred with a neurologist and ENT and referred her for assessment. It turned out she had stage four carcinoma of the parotid gland. She had wasted nine months being treated for TMJ and would have waited another six months if she had not come to our practice for help.

We saw her husband about a year or so later and he reported that she was doing fine and that we literally had saved her life.

I'm not sharing this story to impress you with how great we are, but rather to impress upon you yet again, how *vitally important* it is for you to select the right doctor, have a *thorough* assessment performed and have an *accurate diagnosis* made before instituting treatment.

I hope after reading this book, you will have become a more informed and discerning patient who will no longer be content with a quick-fix solution or a handful of prescriptions.

There are many, many case studies that I could share with you:

· The young lady who had to get out of bed and crawl on the floor into the bathroom every morning because she was in so much pain, who now calls us her "little angels" because she is pain free.

· The fellow who had tried everything to restore his balance and had been unable to find a solution who now is back playing golf and other sports with his balance restored

· The middle-aged lady who had endured severe headaches for her entire adult life, been to numerous neurologists, tried every migraine medication on the market along with Botox injections, hydrocodone and oxycodone all with minimal relief and now leads a happy life free of all these medications

· The wealthy older gentleman who had flown from coast to coast all across the United States in his private jet to seek care for his TMJ pain with the nation's leading experts all to no avail, who is now comfortable, functional and a dear friend of ours

· The young fellow who had undergone two major orthognathic surgeries to reposition his maxilla, still was in severe pain and had a terrible bite relationship and is now (to use his words) delighted with our result and what life holds for him

· The young lady suffering from chronic nerve pain and TMJ disorder barely able to open her mouth or smile without pain who had been to all kinds of specialists and neurologists and no one was able to help her who we discovered had a connective tissue disorder, referred to a rheumatologist, made a TMJ appliance and reduced her trigeminal neuralgia

· The young lady experiencing severe headaches and migraines that lasted for three months twenty four hours a day that now has had a life-changing experience and zero headaches

I could go on and on with case after case and many of them would be compelling for you to read about. I feel so privileged and honored to be able to have impacted their lives in such a positive way. The common thread in all of these cases is – they had been to numerous other health professionals to no avail.

In my opinion, a proper physiological work-up/assessment had not been performed to determine the underlying cause of the pain and dysfunction and instead symptomatic treatment had been offered. They all made progress when the underlying issues were addressed.

However, one case in particular stands out in my mind as most noteworthy, and this is the case I will share with you. The reason this case is so notable is not because of us - but rather because of the remarkable lady who would not give in to her chronic pain, who would not give up on the possibility of improving her quality of life.

I wonder how many of you would have given up hope and accepted a 'life sentence' of pain rather than persisting in looking for an ultimate solution to improve your life. This young lady would not take 'no' for an answer. I'm glad she found us.

Her name is Susan Severino. I asked her how she felt about becoming, "a chapter in my book" and being the sweetheart she is, she felt if her case study helped anyone else who is suffering, to move forward and get free from pain, then allowing me to chronicle her story was worthwhile.

If you have been disappointed in the past by the results of previous attempts to relieve your pain, I hope that Susan's story can serve as an inspiration of what's possible when you do not give in to your present circumstances and accept them as permanent.

Susan presented to our office on October 29th, 2013 for a consultation. She shared with me that she had been dealing with chronic pain for over 4 ½ years and had seen 13 doctors since May 21st, 2009. She stated, "Nothing and no one had been able to help me."

On the *initial history form* that she filled out for us she reported:

· Difficulty to open wide
· Crunching in ears since May 21, 2009
· Bite feels unstable, uncomfortable
· Pain in her ears, neck, head, behind her eyes

· Frequent headaches, neck aches, ear aches, all getting worse

· To cope with the pain she would go to bed

· Had tried hydrocodone, Celebrex, Diclofenac, Etodolac and NSAIDs

· Vestibular symptoms included ears feel stuffy/congested, ringing in ears, often dizzy

· Present symptoms are debilitating and cannot function

Among the 13 doctors she had been to she had received pain management, injections, acupuncture, dry needling, surgery, manipulations and the list goes on. Nothing had worked.

Axially corrected tomograms to show the position and condition of her temporomandibular joints were taken on November 6th, 2013. The images revealed:

· Reduced superior joint space left and right joints
· Flattening on the left condylar head
· Intact lamina dura
· Normal glenoid fossa

A *physiological, neuromuscular work up* was performed on November 19th, 2013. The work up revealed:

Pain scale: Gets as bad as an 8/9 on a scale of 1 – 10. Onset – daily. Nothing relieves the pain

Sleep – wakes up in pain
Appetite – less intake
Physical activity – no physical activity
Relationships – family and friends affected
Emotions – frustration; nothing seems to help
Concentration – focus greatly affected

Other – normal life is influenced by pain

History:

September 1989 – bike accident; flew over the handlebars; hit the pavement with chin

May 21, 2009 – woke up with ear pain and crunching in joint

Head and neck muscle examination:

TMJ capsule – tender
Temporalis Anterior – tender left and right
Medial Pterygoid – painful left and right
Digastric – painful left and right
Sternocleidomastoid – tender left; painful right

Neck range of motion – posterior cranial rotation limited, left/right rotation limited, tilt left/right limited

Shoulder range of motion – normal

Existing Shimbashi: # 9/24 15.5 mm. (Shimbashi is a name given to a particular measurement taken intra-orally that shows the distance gumline to gumline of two selected opposing teeth. For example, if we measure the distance from the gumline of your upper central incisor to the gumline of your lower central incisor when your mouth is closed and your teeth are touching together, we will get a number. The normal range between the two central incisors is somewhere between 17mm. and 21 mm. We also record this measurement between opposing back teeth, but to keep this simple I provided only the front measurement.)

So since Susan's measurement was only 15.5 mm it shows that she was overclosed. Our new target Shimbashi will be 21 mm.

Much of the physiological work-up is accomplished utilizing a computer:

· Computerized mandibular scanning (CMS) tracking the movement, velocity, range of motion and position of the mandible
· Electrosonography (ESG) joint vibrational analysis
· Electromyography (EMG) measurement of muscle function and activity

In order to prevent your eyes from rolling back into your head as you're reading all this, let me try to make sense of this for you. I could write a volume of three books just on the physiology of the head and neck and the various tests we perform. It's not relevant here.

Let it suffice to say that – as a result of four hours of testing, we determined that Susan's jaw was retruded by 3.8 mm and overclosed. In 'people terms' - her bite was positioning her lower jaw too far back and too far up. Her EMGs showed her muscles were, 'on fire' in her existing bite. They could not achieve true rest. The muscles that had to try to stabilize and support the jaw in this position were pooped. Plain worn out.

Diagnosis:

Mal-relationship of her mandible (lower jaw) to her cranium (head) with resulting muscle fatigue and spasm.

We determined where her muscles and joints would optimally like to be positioned if her teeth hadn't gotten in the way. We took a bite registration of the new, improved position.

We had the laboratory create a clear, plastic, removable appliance that fit over Susan's lower teeth. When worn, it allows her to speak, chew, sleep and function all day with her lower jaw and teeth all in the optimal position where her muscles are happy and relaxed.

Therapy:

We delivered this new orthotic to Susan on December 10th, 2013. We TENS'd her for an hour to relax her muscles and then balanced the appliance. We saw her for a follow up appointment two days later. Again we TENS'd her for an hour and balanced the appliance. She reported she was already feeling better.

Susan's next visit was one month later, on January 9th, 2014. At this visit she reported she was 95% better. Not to brag, but in one month's time we accomplished what thirteen other doctors over a period of four and a half years could not - relieve her pain.

It wasn't, "in her head" and she chose not to give up and just, "live with it". When adequate time was taken to determine what the actual underlying cause of the pain was and appropriate steps taken to correct it – the pain went away.

What's the takeaway here? A great lady with a great attitude, plus proper diagnostics, plus proper therapy, equaled success. No magic. Just solid science and an accurate diagnosis. You shouldn't settle for anything less, should you?

Frequently Asked Questions

How do I know if I'm a good candidate for this therapy?

Basic physiology is basic physiology. Muscles are muscles. No matter who we are, our bodies operate according to the same laws of physics and biology. If you have pain or dysfunction as described in the previous chapters, there is an extremely high likelihood you would respond to therapy.

Is the treatment painful?

No, not at all. Most patients find the hour of TENS prior to any minor adjustments being made to their orthotic, extremely relaxing, almost euphoric. The physical therapy appointments utilizing multiple modalities such as ultrasound, cold laser, NuCalm, trigger point muscle relaxation, etc. are all comfortable procedures. Once a patient is in their new appliance, symptoms slowly start to diminish so again, pain is being reduced not increased.

What's wrong with just stopping the symptoms from creating pain?

If the underlying, primary cause of the pain is not addressed and removed – then the muscles, nerves, connective tissue, tendons, ligaments and discs all continue to degenerate and grow progressively worse.

Kicking the can a little further down the road just leaves a bigger mess for the next doctor to have to correct.

What are the warning signs that my headaches are caused by my TMJ?

1. Your jaw clicks or pops.

Any joint in your body should work silently and seamlessly. It should rotate smoothly creating no sound or vibration. If your jaw clicks or pops when you open or close, it's a clear sign that the lower half of the joint (the condyle) is not in the proper position.

Even though the clicking and popping itself does not produce any pain, it's a red flag that the joint is not in the proper position and the muscles that then have to support and stabilize the joint in that improper position are fatigued and they will produce the pain.

2. Your bite feels off.

The only joint in the human body that has 28 teeth stuck between the opening and closing motion of the joint to complicate things, is the TMJ. Every other joint in our body is completely controlled by our muscles; the position of the joint, its movement and range of motion are mediated by muscle.

The exception is our TMJ. This joint has 28 teeth stuck between the opening and closing range of motion. It's the only joint whose position is entirely dictated by where our teeth come together (our bite). Our bite positions our lower jaw which positions our TMJ.

So if your bite feels off or your teeth don't fit together well, there's a good chance your TMJ joints are off also. If they are, then the muscles that have to move, stabilize and support the joints will fatigue and produce pain.

3. You have pain around your forehead, temples, back of head or radiating down your neck.

Ninety percent of pain comes from muscle. If your muscles are not functioning well because of fatigue from supporting one or both of your TMJ joints in an improper position, they produce pain.

This is no different than if you overworked any muscle in your body from too much exercise or work and feel pain later. In the case of your TMJ and headaches the only difference is that it's more subtle and chronic in nature.

4. You have forward head posture.

Your head should be centered over your shoulders. If your head is in front of your shoulders when you're upright, you have 'forward head posture'. This position is related to your bite and your airway.

Your head weighs approximately eight to ten pounds. The further forward off the center axis it is, the more stress and strain it places on your neck muscles and vertebrae. Imagine holding a ten pound bowling ball... the further away from the midline of your body you hold it, the harder it becomes to hold it and support it.

Your neck, back of your head and side of your head can all be in pain from this problem.

5. *You snore.*

Snoring is a red flag that respiration during sleep is disturbed. There are several factors that affect why we snore, but one of the most important is the position of our lower jaw. If our lower jaw is a little too far backward, then our tongue is also further backward since our tongue's position is dictated by where our jaw is.

If the tongue is slightly further back than optimal it vibrates against our soft palate, closes off our airway and we snore. So again, while snoring itself doesn't create headaches, it's another red flag that our lower jaw is too far back and again the muscles that have to support the jaw in an improper position produce the pain.

Additionally, if our respiration during sleep is compromised, we may not be getting enough oxygen and have too much carbon dioxide building up in our bloodstream. This can manifest in 'morning headaches' upon awakening.

What's the main benefit of choosing this treatment over other options?

Unless you just started reading this chapter first, I sincerely hope you can now answer this question yourself. The main benefit is treating the primary cause of the dysfunction and pain – not masking symptoms.

Will the orthotic damage my teeth?

Not at all. It rests gently but securely on top of your lower teeth. No alterations are made to your actual teeth.

Does it matter if I have my family dentist do this for me?

That all depends on who your family dentist is and what their background and training are. Please go re-read chapter 6.

Can I still have regular dental treatment done while I'm in therapy?

Yes, it is recommended to only attend to pressing immediate concerns rather than larger, comprehensive procedures such as crowns, bridges, implants, periodontal surgery, etc.

My dentist made me a nightguard. Doesn't it do the same thing?

No. A night guard is designed to prevent you from grinding your teeth together at night. People who grind their teeth during their sleep can do serious damage to their teeth by wearing down the enamel over time. Once the enamel is ground off the process accelerates and worsens.

Your whole tooth is not made of enamel. It's only on the outer millimeter or so of the tooth. The inner part of the tooth is a material called dentin. It's much softer and more porous. Once the enamel is gone on the biting surface, the dentin wears away much faster so the whole process gets worse and worse.

So the night guard is designed to slow down this destructive process. The thinking goes like this: It's better to wear down and trash a few hundred dollar piece of plastic every few years and replace it, then to continue to damage the teeth themselves. So at least for eight hours out of every twenty-four, you can't do any damage. But here's the problem…

It's not designed or capable of treating or correcting TMJ pain or its related problems such as clicking, jaw popping, headaches, migraines, facial pain, ear pain, dizziness, ringing in the ears, neck pain, etc. It doesn't correct the relationship of the lower jaw to the upper jaw. It doesn't correct the bad bite.

So a night guard is to prevent grinding at night. That's it. It's not for treating complex pain or functional issues of the head and neck. It won't work.

My dentist made me this little device that fits over just my front teeth so they can't touch. She said that would cure my TMJ problems. It helped for a week or two but now I'm back where I started and my teeth are getting sore. What happened?

The device your dentist made is called an NTI. They merely take a mould of the upper and lower teeth and send a prescription to a dental laboratory asking them to make an NTI. That's all that's necessary.

So the NTI is very popular because it requires no advanced study and training to utilize it. The average general or cosmetic dentist has little interest in treating complex pain and TMJ functional issues of the head and neck. That's not what they deal with on a regular basis, but they still want to try to help their patients and not have to refer them out to a TMJ specialist. It's quick and cheap to fabricate.

That's all fine except the NTI, if worn for an extended period of time, can cause an 'open bite.' That's when our back teeth hit together and the front ones are wide apart and don't touch at all. The NTI is acceptable as a 'quick-fix' however there are better 'quick fixes' in our opinion and it can help for a few days or weeks because it prevents the teeth from coming together.

It helps to temporarily shut down the action of the masseter and pterygoid muscles that may be contributing to the pain. If you have one, do not wear it for an extended period of time, such as months. It can eventually open up your bite and will not permanently cure your TMJ pain and problem.

The vast majority of our profession just does not treat advanced, complex TMJ problems on a daily basis. It's not their "thing." So an NTI can be an ok quick-fix, but in my opinion should not be relied on to permanently correct your temporomandibular joint dysfunction and the associated pain.

I've already been to several other doctors and TMJ specialists and no one seems to be really able to help me. Why is this so hard to treat?

Jaw pain, clicking, popping joints and limitation in opening are relatively easy to identify as a TMJ disorder. A dentist should be your first stop. However headaches, migraines, ear congestion, vertigo, tinitis and other diffuse head and neck pain are not so easily identified and may be treated by other health professionals as a different condition. Often, an actual diagnosis is never made and instead drugs are prescribed to provide symptomatic relief.

The key is to make a proper diagnosis. From the diagnosis the correct treatment options to improve or correct your condition can be made.

If you suffer from head and neck pain, headaches, migraines, vertigo or tinnitus and have not seen *any* health professional yet, it certainly is reasonable to start with your family physician to assess your condition and rule out any other serious condition such as cancer, tumors, cysts, neurological disorders, Menier's disease, arthritis, etc.

However, if you have already been to numerous doctors, been treated for numerous maladies with no result – then the advice in this book can serve you well.

Will I need surgery?

There are indications for surgery; however surgery is the means of last resort for headaches, migraines or TMJ dysfunction. Since ninety percent of pain originates in the muscles, there are many options to relieve pain and improve function without having to resort to surgery.

Please understand, surgery is the correct option and sometimes the only option depending on what the medical condition is. I certainly am not against surgery when indicated.

But when it comes to treating headaches, migraines and TMJ dysfunction, there are other more conservative solutions that can be utilized first.

Can I have Botox?

Sure. Botox works. It temporarily freezes the muscles that cause the headache and migraine pain. However, it needs to be redone approximately every three months. So ask yourself how many times do you desire to get over thirty injections per treatment stuck in your head?

It's a quick-fix approach. A valid quick-fix, but nevertheless, a quick-fix.

*** Well, I've gone over the questions we get asked most often. But what about the questions we *never* get asked? What about the questions you don't even know to ask? As my mentor Dr. Bill Dickerson would always say, "You don't know what you don't know." Truer words were never spoken.

Here is the one question, in my opinion, that's the most important of all:

Ok, I know I have a problem. But what happens if I just do nothing?

Well, it depends on what your actual problem is. Every action has consequences. So does every failure to act.

There's the physical component we've discussed in detail. If something in our body is being assaulted, if something is degenerating, then the consequences of doing nothing allows our body to continue to deteriorate.

We're already fighting degeneration just from the mere act of aging. But there's a more insidious problem at work here. How do we feel knowing that our body isn't right, that we are living with constant pain? The emotional, psychological toll is in some ways even greater.

I don't want to be presumptuous enough to tell you how to live your life – but I can share with you that so many, many people I have treated over the years were beaten down, living a diminished life, from their maladies. This isn't how we're supposed to function and feel. A better life awaits.

This is my belief. It's why I do what I do. My belief is that people can be happier, more productive and more successful when they are free from pain or disease. Since I have the ability to help people and see the change in their lives when they're healed ... there is nothing else I'd rather do.

Remember I said it depends what your problem is? People don't generally die from headaches, migraines and TMJ dysfunction. But, if you have undiagnosed obstructive sleep apnea that we also previously discussed... you *could* die if you do nothing. Stroke and heart attack are an ever-present risk.

So either way, the entire purpose of writing, 'Break Away' was to give you the knowledge and motivation to move forward with getting the appropriate care to get whole and get healthy again.

The second most important question:

How much better can your life be if you *do* take action?

Conclusion

WELL, WE'VE COVERED a lot of ground. I don't think you have quite enough knowledge to take over my practice yet, but I hope you now know enough 'to be dangerous'. I've thrown a lot at you in a very short period of time.

We discussed pain and its origins and outcome. We talked about the many faces of TMJ and how easily it is misdiagnosed resulting in many of our symptoms being interpreted as something else. We talked about the cause and effect of temporomandibular joint dysfunction and took the mystery out of why we hurt.

We discussed headaches and migraines in detail. We spoke about the shortcomings of the pharmaceutical industry and the health profession's dirty little secret of treating symptoms. We uncovered the fallacy of a quick-fix mentality. We went over all the various treatment options available to you. We discussed the best treatment option and why it's best.

I even gave you a few thought-provoking questions along the way to examine your own attitudes toward pain and fear. We went over a case study together to try to show you that you should not accept what a few doctors may have already told you about just 'living with your pain' at face value - and instead should push on undiscouraged, until you have your solution.

We answered some of the commonly asked questions. And now ... it's time to conclude.

So let me ask you this: do I wind up on a shelf in your home with other books, quickly forgotten? Do you say, "That was very interesting and informative." *or* - did I break through to you and give you a wake up call?

Did we kick down some doors and break some windows to let some light in and show you what is *really* holding you back from becoming pain free? Do you now understand the true cause of your pain – the root cause?

Will you change what you've accepted up until now as acceptable care and advice? This is your defining moment. What are you going to fight for? Are you now determined to find the actual solution to your chronic pain?

We are incredible human beings with an amazing capacity to heal. The question isn't whether this is true. The question is whether or not you believe it. I sure hope so.

I'm here to tell you that you can live your life, being your best - being free from the chronic pain of headaches, migraines and TMJ dysfunction. I've done my very best to arm you with the necessary information to 'BREAK AWAY' from old, ineffective methods of treatment and be able to move forward to get the proper help.

So my time to work with you has now come to a close. Now it's your turn to take action and don't stop until you're healed. *You can do this.* This is *your time* on this earth. Your time to be healthy, happy and thrive. Make the most of it.

The H.E.A.L. Formula™

HELP yourself - take control of your outcome. Don't accept chronic pain as a life sentence and stop taking pills to mask symptoms. When you improve your health, the lives of those around you improve also – not just you. There's more love, happiness and fun for everyone.

EVERYTHING is connected. The teeth. The joints. The tendons. The ligaments. The jaw. The head. The neck. The muscles. They all have to work together in harmony to not produce pain.

ALIGN the jaw. Align the bite. When everything is aligned, the muscles are happy. And happy muscles do not create pain.

LEARN about and utilize the new methods for successfully treating chronic headaches, migraines and TMJ without medication. I challenge you to think differently about the true cause of your chronic pain.

Now you have an opportunity to discard your old, ineffective beliefs and with your newfound knowledge of the physiology of pain, seek effective solutions. The best time to have done this was when your pain first began. The second best time - *is right now.*

Acknowledgments

WE ALL ARE the product of many people who come into our lives... some for a short period of time, and others whom we have relationships with for decades. I would like to give my heart-felt thanks to the people who have helped make this book possible.

First and foremost, I would like to thank my family. My beautiful and amazing wife of forty-two years, Rhona, who has been by my side through thick and thin and always encouraged me to share my knowledge with the world. As the old saying goes, "behind every successful man there's a great woman" and that's absolutely the case here.

I want to thank my beautiful children, Jennifer and Jeffrey, who both are an inspiration to me and an example of overcoming illness to ultimately go on to lead healthy, productive lives. By the way, Jeffrey, who has mad skills as a graphic artist and designer, created the cover for this book. Very cool.

There are many teachers and mentors who come into our lives. Some are terrible. Some are good. And a few are great. And - if we're really lucky - there may be that special individual, who through patience, guidance and support may completely change our life and career.

I was lucky enough to have this type of mentor and friend. His name is Dr. Bill Dickerson and he is the founder and CEO of the Las Vegas Institute for Advanced Dental Studies. I would not be the dentist I am today, or possess the advanced knowledge to successfully treat and positively impact so many patients' lives if it were not for Bill's unrelenting commitment to our profession and education and the amazing think tank he has created. He represents the very best of what excellence in health care is truly about.

I'd be remiss if I didn't thank my talented assistant and dear friend of thirteen years, Angie Nester who has been my right arm and left arm in the clinic. We have both learned so much from each other. Dr. Omer Reed, another wonderful mentor, calls people like Angie and I a "care pair". I don't think there's a better "care pair" anywhere because of this great lady.

And lastly, whether you feel it is hokey or not, I want to thank the Good Lord for blessing me with such a wonderful life filled with the greatest of friends, family and patients to love and honor.

All of my talents come from the Big Guy upstairs and I know it and give thanks every day for all the blessings He's bestowed upon me during my brief stay on this earth. If I can make this world a better place, even by just a little, because of the knowledge and care I have to share with people, then my time on this earth will have been well spent.

God Bless.

About the Author

Dr. Fred Abeles is known as one of the most sought after TMJ experts in the United States. He's famous for getting results where all others have failed and getting those results without the use of surgery, needles or drugs.

Patients from the US, Canada and abroad travel to the Atlanta Center for TMJ for Dr. Abeles' care. He is the Clinical Instructor and Regional Director for the Las Vegas Institute for Advanced Dental Studies - one of the most prestigious post-graduate teaching centers in the world today.

Dr. Abeles has been featured on NBC and CBS, consults with leading dental manufacturers on the development of new dental products, been on the cover of the profession's biggest magazines and instructed dentists throughout the United States and Canada on state-of-the-art techniques for treating headaches and temporomandibular joint dysfunction.

Dr. Abeles is an accomplished jazz and concert pianist. He's performed for three U.S. Presidents, appeared with Jerry Lewis, Vic Damone and numerous Hollywood celebrities. He's been a guest artist with the Atlanta Pops Symphony Orchestra and still entertains at charity events in the Atlanta Area.

He resides in Atlanta with his beautiful wife of forty-two years, Rhona, and his two children, Jennifer and Jeffrey.